A Companion to Homeopathic Studies

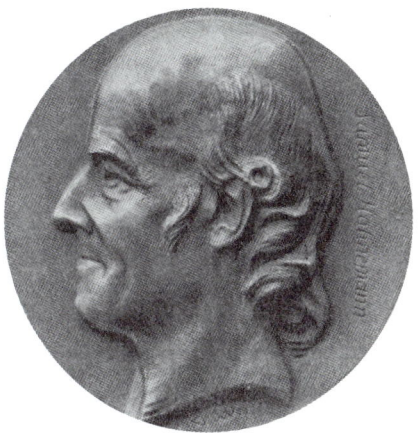

Bronze plaque of Samuel Hahnemann, founder of homeopathy, by the sculptor David d'Angers, 1839.

Other works by the same author:
Homoeopathy for Physicians
The Dental Prescriber
Die homöopathische Verordnung in der zahnärtzlichen Praxis
The Biochemic Handbook
Handbuch der homöopathischen Gewebesalze
The Traveller's Prescriber
The Infinitesimal Dose
A Textbook of Dental Homoeopathy★
The World Travellers' Manual of Homoeopathy★
Homöopathisches Reisehandbuch
Handboek Homeopathie voor de Wereldreiziger
Homoeopathic Remedies – An International Handbook
The Complementary Formulary
A Letter on Medical Electricity
A New Physics of Homeopathy
★*also available in Japanese*

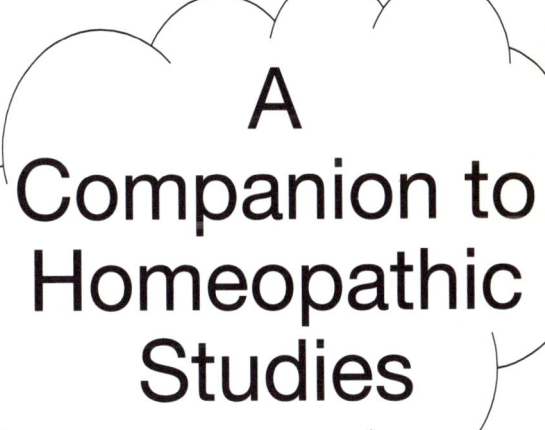

A Companion to Homeopathic Studies

Dr Colin B. Lessell
MB, BS, BDS, MRCS, LRCP, DDFHom,
FBHomDA, HonFHMA

Index compiled by
Ann Griffiths

SAFFRON WALDEN
THE C.W. DANIEL COMPANY LIMITED

First published in the United Kingdom by
by The C.W. Daniel Company Limited
1 Church Path, Saffron Walden,
Essex, CB10 1JP, United Kingdom

© Colin B. Lessell 2003

ISBN 0 85207 363 1

The author has asserted his rights under the Copyright Design and Patent Act 1988 (and under any comparable provision of any comparable law in any jurisdiction whatsoever) to be identified as the author of this work.

So far as may legally effectively be provided no liability of any kind or nature whatsoever, whether in negligence, under statute, or otherwise, is accepted by the authors or the publishers for the accuracy or safety of any of the information or advice contained in, or in any way relating to any part of the content of, this book.

All rights reserved. No part of this publication may be reproduced, stored in a retrieval system, or transmitted in any form or by any means, electronic, mechanical, photocopying, recording, or otherwise, without the prior permission of the copyright holder.

The author wishes to thank the publishers for their kind permission to incorporate edited material from *A Textbook of Dental Homoeopathy*, 1st/2nd editions, 1995/2000.

Produced in association with Book Production Consultants, plc,
25–27 High Street, Chesterton, Cambridge, CB4 1ND
Text designed and typeset by Ward Partnership, Saffron Walden, Essex
Printed and bound in Great Britain by
St Edmundsbury Press, Bury St Edmunds, Suffolk

'No great discovery was ever made without a bold guess.'

Sir Isaac Newton (1642–1726)
Quoted in W. I. B. Beveridge (1950)
The Art of Scientific Investigation.

Contents

Figures ix
Introduction xi

1 Thinking about how remedies are selected 1

Introduction – More about cause and cure – What is the 'simillimum'? – How are remedies selected? – Constitutional aspects of pathological prescribing – The 'pathological simillimum' – Constitutional prescribing – What is a repertory? – Repertorization of thermal sensitivity – The materia medica – What are leading symptoms? – Prescription by causation – Using a therapeutic index, repertory and materia medica – What is a miasm? – What is 'Hering's Law'? – Potencies and frequency of repetition – What is a 'similior'?

2 Thinking about how remedies are made 24

Introduction – Pharmaceutical objectives – Scales of serial dilution – Manufacture of LMs – Mother tinctures – Diluents – Impurities – Types of energization – Classical energization: succussion – Classical energization: trituration – Fluxion – Bubbling and prepotentization – Electromagnetic energization – Boiling – Erasure of imprinting – Preparatory vessels – Medication of solid forms.

3 Thinking about how remedies work 72

Introduction 73

Part One
Receptor-mediated action of remedies (Type I action) 77
Pharmacodynamic docking and locking – Agonism versus antagonism – Physicochemical concepts in agonism and antagonism

– Van der Waals' forces and the Casimir effect – Summation of geometric conformation – Substitution with the field concept – Remedies as fields – Homeopathic blocking or shielding – Allergenic isopathy –Viral remedies (viral nosodes) – Homeopathic blocking of therapeutic drugs – Homeopathic action of material doses of drugs – Duration of action of potentized remedies – Explanation of the actions of *Arnica* and *Euphrasia* – Explanation of the actions of *Mercurius* and *Arsenicum*.

Part Two
Non-receptor-mediated action of remedies
(Type II action) 93
Fundamental ideas – Further concepts of disease – Geometric concepts – Multiple subsets in chronic disease – Intermediate states – Electromagnetic radiation remedies – Conclusion.

4 Thinking about dosage and related matters 103

Introduction – Mother tinctures – Liquid potencies – Dosage of liquid and solid forms – Triturated material – Potency and therapeutic response – Dose repetition – Storage of solid forms – Precautions in taking remedies – Adverse effects of potentized remedies – Administration of remedies to breastfed babies – Complex prescriptions – Placebos.

Glossary of physiochemical terms   121

Sources of information and supply   127

References   129

Index   131

Figures

1.1	Title page of Samuel Hahnemann's first formal enunciation of the homeopathic method, published in 1796 in the *Journal der practischen Arzneykunde und Wundarzneykunst* (*Journal of Practical Pharmaceutics and Surgery*), edited by Hufeland in Jena, Germany.	4
1.2	Vials, globules and a leather remedy wallet. From the pricelist of the Dr Willmar Schwabe Pharmacy, Leipzig, *c.* 1900.	8
1.3	German domestic remedy chest and a traveller's kit. From the pricelist of the Dr Willmar Schwabe Pharmacy, Leipzig, *c.* 1900.	17
2.1	Title page of the first edition of Hahnemann's *Organon*, 1810 (Dresden, Arnold).	27
2.2	Samuel Hahnemann. From a daguerrotype taken 30 September 1841 in Paris.	28
2.3	Capillary tube for regulating drops. From the pricelist of the Dr Willmar Schwabe Pharmacy, Leipzig, *c.* 1900.	32
2.4	York Glass Company's percolator. For the production of mother tinctures. London, *British Homoeopathic Pharmacopoeia*, 1882.	37
2.5	Herb and plant press. German illustration, *c.* 1920.	38
2.6	The three standard diluents of homeopathic pharmacy. 1: Water. 2: Ethanol. 3: Lactose.	39
2.7	Glucose isomers.	41
2.8	Methods of energization.	47
2.9	Somolinos Mechanical Succussion Apparatus. From the pricelist of La Farmacia Homeopática de Don Cesáreo Martín Somolinos, Madrid, 1866.	48
2.10	Benoît Mure Succussion Machine, *c.* 1838. The first mechanical succussion apparatus.	49
2.11	Anthroposophical succussion. (Photograph by courtesy of Weleda UK Ltd., Ilkeston.)	51

2.12	Distillation plant for the production of spirits. Homeopathic Central Pharmacy of Dr Willmar Schwabe, Leipzig, c. 1920.	52
2.13	Benoît Mure Triturator, c. 1838.	53
2.14	Hewitt Mechanical Triturator. From the pricelist of La Farmacia Homeopática de Don Cesáreo Martin Somolinos, Madrid, 1866.	54
2.15	Trituration Machine. Homeopathic Central Pharmacy of Dr Willmar Schwabe, Leipzig, c. 1920.	56
2.16	Microscopy of handmade trituration of *Cuprum metallicum* (copper) D1. Magnification: 180 ×.	57
2.17	Microscopy of *Cuprum metallicum* (copper) D1 after 60 minutes of trituration with the Dr Willmar Schwabe machine.	58
2.18	Microscopy of trituration.	58
2.19	The Skinner Fluxion Centesimal Potentizer/Attenuator, c. 1878.	64
2.20	Benoît Mure Vacuum Device, c. 1838.	65
2.21	Perdrisat-Nebel Automatic Potentizer, early twentieth century.	67
2.22	Weber Potentizer, nineteenth century.	68
3.1	Title page of Hahnemann's early description of the use of *Belladonna* and other drugs in infinitesimal doses, 1801 (Berlin, Hufeland's journal).	75
3.2	Pen sketches by Hahnemann, displaying an interest in succussive blows.	76
3.3	The basic coarse geometric principles involved in homeopathic pharmacodynamics and drug–receptor docking.	83
3.4	An abstract representation of homeopathic shielding using blocks.	86
3.5	An abstract representation of the four basic theoretical geometrical interactions of a remedy field {pF★} with a subset {pE★} using blocks.	97
3.6	Bottles of homeopathic *Chamomilla* for domestic use. Dr Willmar Schwabe Pharmacy, Leipzig, c. 1900.	102
4.1	English advertisement for homeopathic remedies, 1875. From the *British Homoeopathic Medical and Pharmaceutical Directory*.	105
4.2	Manufacture of globules and pillules. German illustration, c. 1920.	110

Introduction

There are three types of homeopathic student: the plodder, the jogger and the *thinker*. The plodder dully plods along, slavishly learning according to rote, and regurgitating facts with the precision of a mynah bird. The jogger enthusiastically jogs through as many courses, lectures and conferences as are available, seldom having time to think or regurgitate. The *thinker*, however, worries profoundly about the very foundations of homeopathy, and spends more time in the pub with a fist under the chin (sometimes his own). This is a book for the *thinker* – not the plodder, or the jogger.

Of course, you may not think of yourself as much of a *thinker*, merely because your thoughts have come to nought. But you really are a *thinker* if you think about any of the following (especially during a boring lecture):

- How remedy selection can be simplified
- How therapeutic efficacy survives repeated dilution
- Why impurities make little difference to the resultant remedy
- How remedies are really made
- How different approaches to manufacture lead to different therapeutic properties
- The chemistry of substances which can 'remember' others
- Historical variations in processing
- How remedies work
- How material doses of drugs can act homeopathically
- The sites of action of remedies on the living organism
- The action of the living organism on remedies
- The basis for idiosyncratic responses to therapy
- How the different scales of dilution can be compared
- How to prescribe for a tee-total vegan with sucrose intolerance.

So hopefully, this is a book for you, containing most of the answers to all those questions you might have put to yourself or others, without gaining a satisfactory response. In fact, it is intended to be a true complement to your studies, rather than a complete textbook in its own right. In order to meet the needs of students of all levels (from beginner to post-graduate), persuasions (physician, non-physician, pharmacist, manqué, etc.) and routes of attack (full-time, part-time, bed-time, etc.), I have included some very basic material within the text. But I venture that even the established practitioner may benefit from reading Chapters 2–4, whilst perhaps finding the odd gem also in Chapter 1.

Any commentary on the physicochemical nature of remedies has been extracted, extended and crystallized from *A New Physics of Homeopathy* (Lessell, 2002), to which the reader with further interest may care to refer in due course. Any mathematics contained in the text, though novel in application, is of the simplest nature. Those who find the idea of 'sets' and 'subsets' somewhat daunting might be reassured that a 'set' is merely a list of objects. Hence, a shopping list is really a set composed of subsets, albeit a somewhat costly one these days. Thus, {cheese, bread, wine} is a set, of which {wine} is a subset. Sets and subsets may be added or subtracted just like ordinary numbers, e.g.:

$$\{\text{cheese, bread, wine}\} - \{\text{wine}\} = \{\text{cheese, bread}\}.$$

This should be a sobering thought, if nothing else, for those about to embark on this 'crash course'.

Colin Lessell
Kleine Schweiz

Failure in treatment more often depends on the selection of a totally inappropriate remedy, rather than an incorrect potency. Failure also results from the inability of the practitioner to realize that homeopathic treatment is unlikely to be the best initial approach (e.g. in a case of nutritional deficiency). Indeed, we might say that a good homeopath knows when not to use homeopathy, whilst a bad one uses it all the time and without exception. Upon a similar basis, of course, we might also judge the orthodox practitioner.

1
Thinking about how remedies are selected

Introduction

This chapter gives a concise outline of the methodology of homeopathic remedy selection, and is mainly intended for those relatively new to the subject. Fortunately, there is sufficient flexibility in prescribing to enable even the beginner to produce tolerably good results in relatively straightforward cases.

As is well known, homeopathy is based on the **Law of Similars** ('Let likes be treated with likes', if you like), also known as the **Similia Principle**. This tells us that where a drug is capable of producing a disease syndrome in a healthy subject, then it may be used to treat a disease syndrome of similar character in the sick (in which case it is termed a **remedy**). Hence, the use of *Belladonna* in scarlet fever, from the correspondence of the toxic effects of the drug with those of the disease. The modern use of dilutions of food substances to treat food intolerance is merely a 'rediscovery' of the same principle, as is the case of the 'rediscovery' of the notion of holistic medicine by the orthodox profession.

With regard to nomenclature and labelling, unless determined otherwise by the practitioner, each dispensed remedy should bear its full Latin name (e.g. *Aconitum napellus*, *Natrum muriaticum*, *Phosphorus*) – or an easily recognizable abbreviation (e.g. *Aconite*, *Nat. mur.*, *Phos.*) – plus its therapeutic strength, or **potency**, as it is termed (e.g. *Aconite 6c*, *Nat. mur. D12*), the meaning of which will be explained in due course (see Chapter 2, *Scales of serial dilution*). The survival of Latin within homeopathy means that any homeopath or homeopathic pharmacist can recognize the product instantly in every part of the world. Indeed, most remedies have a Latin name, the main exceptions being some remedies of relatively modern incorporation within the materia medica (e.g. *Gunpowder*). Certainly, with such remedies as *Medorrhinum* (gonococcal nosode) and *Lueticum* (syphilitic nosode), the use of romanized jargon is a valid deceit in the case of the squeamish patient. Furthermore, neither the latinization of most of the medicines (or **remedies**, as we prefer to term them), nor the apparently bizarre nature of some of them, should deter the enquiring mind from further investigation. The remedy *Berlin Wall* (which, were it not for the decline in the Classics, might have been called *Murus transversarius Berolini*) is one particular example of a remedy most peculiar.

More about cause and cure

The picture of disease or 'dis-ease' induced by the action of a 'drug' (i.e. a medicine or poison) is termed its **pathogenesis**. It includes both psychological and physical objective and subjective symptoms, and pathological and physiological changes. The pathogenesis is established by recording the effects generated by the drug when it is administered either accidentally or intentionally. An important type of intentional administration is the so-called homeopathic **experimental proving**, where a drug is administered to a number of *healthy* human volunteers, who subsequently document the changes experienced. The drug is administered either in a crude form, or as an attenuated homeopathic preparation. **Sporadic or clinical proving** may also occur during actual treatment, when the patient generates new and unusual symptoms related to the medicine given (see Chapter 4, *Adverse effects of potentized remedies*). The results of **provings** (experimental and clinical), together with the symptomatic and pathological details recorded in cases of accidental or malicious poisoning (viz. toxicology), constitute the basis of the homeopathic **materia medica**. When you read about symptoms or diseases in works of homeopathic materia medica, you must realize that it is implied that the relevant substance may either *cause* or *cure* the listed abnormalities, according to circumstances and dosage. Remedies of wide clinical application (e.g. *Sulphur*, *Pulsatilla*, *Mercurius solubilis*) are called **polychrests**. We shall examine the structure of the materia medica later on in this chapter, and discuss how it has been (and *is being*) modified in the light of clinical experience.

What is the 'simillimum'?

The closer the similarity between the documented pathogenesis of the drug and the disease picture of a particular patient, the more likely that the drug will effect a cure in that patient. Drugs which

Journal

der

practischen

Arzneykunde

und

Wundarzneykunst

herausgegeben

von

C. W. Hufeland

der Arzneykunde ordentlichem Lehrer
zu Iena.

Zweyter Band Drittes Stück.

Iena,
in der academischen Buchhandlung
1796.

Figure 1.1
Essay on a new principle for ascertaining the curative powers of drugs, with a few glances at those hitherto employed. Title page (right) of Samuel Hahnemann's

IV.

Verfuch über ein neues Prinzip zur Auffindung der Heilkräfte der Arzneifubftanzen, nebft einigen Blicken auf die bisherigen.

von

D. Samuel Hahnemann.

Zu Anfange diefes Iahrhunderts that man, vorzüglich die Akademie der Wiffenfchaften zu Paris, der Scheidekunft die unverdiente Ehre an, fie als Entdeckerin der Heilkräfte der Arzneien, vorzüglich der Pflanzen, in Verfuchung zu führen. Man trieb die Pflanzen in Deftillirgefäfsen gewöhnlich ohne Waffer, mit Feuergewalt und erzwang dadurch — aus den giftigften wie aus den unfchuldigften — ziemlich einerley Produkte. Waffer, Säure, brenzliche Oele, Kohle — und

first formal enunciation of the homeopathic method, published in 1796 in the *Journal der practischen Arzneykunde und Wundarzneykunst (Journal of Practical Pharmaceutics and Surgery)*, edited by Hufeland in Jena, Germany (left).

exhibit such a close correspondence are said to be **homeopathic** to the disease. The drug which is felt to have the greatest symptomatic and pathological correspondence is termed the **simillimum** (from the Latin, 'the most similar'), a more expansive definition of which will be provided below. For the moment, let it be emphasized that the selection of the simillimum rests not only on the orthodox diagnostic entity (i.e. the name of the disease) but also, in many instances, on the individualized objective and subjective symptomatology (signs and symptoms respectively, as they are otherwise termed). Such symptomatic pictures may vary considerably between cases of disease within the same diagnostic category (e.g. influenza), each case requiring a different simillimum. In other situations (such as the common traumatic bruise or dental abscess), the symptomatic response is more uniform, and the choice of a possible simillimum more limited, and hence simpler.

How are remedies selected?

Remedies may have a generalized or **constitutional** therapeutic effect, or a more restricted action on particular pathologies (or biochemical dysfunctions). The latter is termed their **pathological action**, and, in this respect, the use of a **therapeutic index** is most appropriate (e.g. Lessell, 2001). This is an alphabetical index of diseases and syndromes classified in the orthodox or common manner. A number of different homeopathic (and other) treatments are given under each diagnostic entity (see also below, *What is a 'similior'?*).

Although sometimes we are fortunate in having remedies which exhibit an exact correspondence with a particular orthodox category (e.g. *Hepar sulph.* in the subacute/chronic dental abscess), in many cases, in order to prescribe satisfactorily, the objective and subjective symptoms (signs and symptoms) individually manifested by the patient must be taken into consideration. For example, although *Chamomilla* is almost routinely prescribed for infantile teething, it may fail in cases with excessive salivation, where *Mercurius solubilis* is better indicated. Even the character of a pain may be of some relevance: throbbing, stabbing, burning, crushing, and so on. The 'laterality' of the symptoms may also determine the selection of the remedy – *Sanguinaria* being more commonly indicated in right-sided migraine and *Spigelia* in that involving the left side of the head. **Concomitant symptoms**, remote from the area of pathology, such as the occurrence of extreme restlessness with cold sores, may indicate one remedy rather than another (in this case, *Rhus toxicodendron*).

Also often warranting consideration are things or circumstances which make a complaint or a person better or worse. These are termed **modalities**. In this respect, homeopaths have borrowed the symbols < and > from mathematics, meaning 'less than' and 'greater than' respectively. In homeopathy, however, they are taken to mean 'worse/worse for' (<, lessening of health) and 'better/better for' (>, increase in health). Hence, 'toothache > cold water in mouth' means that cold rinses help the toothache. Modalities may be classified as follows.

1. *Thermal*: < or > heat or cold.
2. *Climatic*: e.g. < or > rain, storms, wind, snow, humidity, change in the weather.
3. *Thermoclimatic*: e.g. humid heat, cold winds, hot rooms.
4. *Periodic* or *Time*: e.g. < after midnight, between 4 and 8p.m., monthly, annually, in summer.
5. *Kinetic* or *Positional*: e.g. < or > movement, staying still, descent, lying on left side.
6. *Nervous*: e.g. < mental exertion, sunlight, strong odours, touch.

Remember that modalities can apply to the person in general as well as to any presenting complaint. Sometimes they appear paradoxical. For example, generally < cold, but headache > cold, suggests *Arsenicum album*.

Constitutional aspects of pathological prescribing

Experienced prescribers often utilize an assessment of the **general** or **constitutional** aspects of the patient to assist them in the

b) Apotheken mit Streukügelchen.

1. **Apotheken** mit F-Zylinder

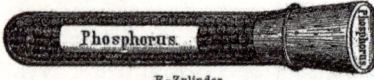

F-Zylinder.

a) in einfach poliertem Kasten mit 12   24   32   48 Mitteln
   ℳ 4,—   6,50   8,50   10,50,

b) in polierten Nussbaumkästen
   mit 60   84   105   120   132   152   180   252   312 Mitteln
   ℳ 17,—   22,50   27,—   30,—   33,—   37,50   44,—   62,—   76,—.

2. **Apotheken** mit O-Zylinder in feinen Nussbaumkästen mit Messingbeschlag mit 12   24   36   48   60   120 Mitteln
   ℳ 17,—   25,—   32,50   40,—   47,—   86,—.

3. **Apotheken** mit P-Zylinder und 3 äusserlichen Mitteln zu 25 g in feinen Nussbaumkästen mit Messingbeschlag
   mit 12   24   36   48   60 Mitteln
   ℳ 19,—   25,—   30,—   35,—   40,—.

4. **Verbesserte Apotheken** mit FF-Zylindern und F-Zylindern in eleganten polierten Nussbaumkästen

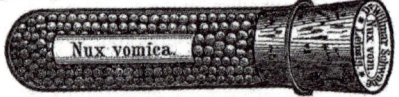

FF-Zylinder.

mit 44   64   88   105   120   132   152   180   204   252   312 M.
ℳ 14,—   19,—   24,—   28,—   32,—   34,—   40,—   46,—   52,—   64,—   80,—.

Die Hauptmittel befinden sich im FF-Zylinder, die weniger gebrauchten im F-Zylinder.

5. **Apotheken** mit 5 Gramm-Flaschen
   a) in Pappkästen mit 8   12   14   20   25 Mitteln
      ℳ 4,50   6,—   6,50   8,50   10,—,
   b) in Nussbaumkästen mit 12   18   24   32   40 Mitteln
      ℳ 7,50   10,—   13,—   16,—   19,50
      mit 50   60   84   105   120   150   200   312 Mitteln
      ℳ 23,50   27,50   37,—   47,—   52,50   64,—   86,50   132,—.

6. **Apotheken** (Nussbaum) mit 25, 15 und 5 Gramm-Flaschen
   mit 25   42   49   66   85   108   134   152   180   204   312 M.
   ℳ 16,50   24,—   28,—   35,50   45,—   56,—   77,—   81,—   96,—   107,—   151,—.

Figure 1.2

Vials, globules and a leather remedy wallet. From the pricelist of the Dr Willmar Schwabe Pharmacy, Leipzig, c. 1900.

7. **Apotheken** in Schrankform (Eiche oder Nussbaum) in 25, 15
und 5 Gramm-Flaschen mit 42   66   85 Mitteln
                      ℳ 34,50 47,—   65,—.
8. **Taschen- und Reise-Apotheken**
a) in G-Zylindern:

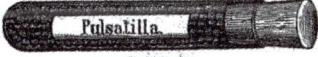

G-Zylinder.

1. einfache   mit 6   12   24   40   60   80 Mitt.
   (Leinw.-Etuis) ℳ 2,25 3,75 6,50 10,— 15,— 19,—,

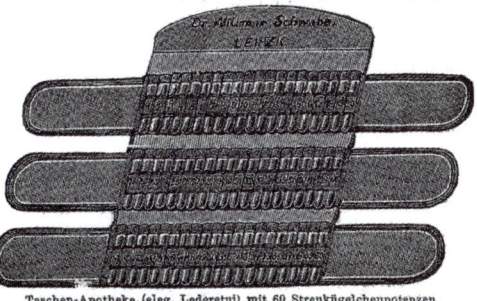

Taschen-Apotheke (eleg. Lederetui) mit 60 Streukügelchenpotenzen.

2. elegante (Leder-Etuis mit Nickelschloss)
   mit 6 12   24   32   40   60   80   100   120   150 Mittl.
   ℳ 3,— 5,— 8,— 10,— 12,50 18,50 24,— 30,— 35,— 43,—,
b) in Schrauben-Zylindern:
   einfache Ausstattung mit 12   24   32   40   60 Mitteln
                        ℳ 6,— 10,50 13,50 17,— 24,50,
   elegante Ausstattung „ 7,— 12,— 16,— 19,50 28,50.
3. Brusttaschen-Etui mit 18 Mitteln, Zylinder EE ℳ 10,—.

c) Apotheken mit Tabletten,
nur als Taschen-Apotheken,
a) einfache Ausstattung mit 12   20   24   30   40   60 Mitt.
                        ℳ 4,50 7,— 8,— 10,— 12,50 18,50;
b) elegante Ausstattung „ 6,— 9,— 10,50 12,50 16,— 22,50.

prescription of an appropriate remedy. For example, *Natrum muriaticum* (*Nat. mur.*) is better suited to a *hot* individual (feels generally < heat) than a chilly one (feels generally > heat). *Sepia*, however, is the opposite. Therefore, in the preventative treatment of cold sores, *Nat. mur.* will be better indicated for the hot woman, and *Sepia* for the chilly one. This is an example of the concept of **susceptible typology**, which essentially means that a certain type or person is sensitive to the action of a particular remedy or group of remedies.

Extending this concept, does this mean that *Nat. mur.* will have no effect on the prevention of cold sores in a chilly person? This might be so; but, more likely, it will exert some effect, but less than it would in a hot type. The patient's general constitution (which includes such parameters as thermal sensitivity, bodily conformation, colouring, pathological predispositions and personality) thus determines, in part, the efficacy of the pathological remedy. *Hepar sulph.*, which almost routinely alleviates subacute or chronic dental abscesses in the majority, is actually most efficacious (i.e. swiftest in action) in those individuals who are flabby, chilly, hypersensitive to pain and easily angered. In other words, this is the 'susceptible typology' for *Hepar sulph.*, and the individual in whom it is manifest is said to be a '*Hepar sulph.* type'. The constitution is named after a remedy to which it significantly corresponds. Similarly, we may talk of '*Phosphorus*', '*Pulsatilla*', '*Sulphur*', '*Calcarea fluorica*', '*Nat. mur.*', and many other 'types'.

The 'pathological simillimum'

The **pathological simillimum** is the remedy best indicated in terms of the individual symptomatology of the patient with regard to the presenting complaint – though sometimes with some partial consideration of the general or constitutional aspects of the case. It is *not*, in view of what has been said, the *only* remedy which will act on the pathology. There is, thus, a certain leeway in homeopathic prescribing, and a remedy that is only partially indicated may still exert a certain beneficial effect. Hence, even when the most theoretically ideal remedy (the simillimum) is unavailable, a secondary remedy may often be selected to great effect (see below, *What is a 'similior'?*).

It should be emphasized that, whereas homeopaths place great emphasis on individual symptomatology, the main action of the chosen pathological remedy is on the pathology itself. There is, however, some evidence (viz. its speed of action) that *Arnica* has some limited analgesic effect in cases of bruising or crushing.

Constitutional prescribing

Constitutional prescribing implies prescription based mainly on the 'general' aspects of the patient, rather than those related to the presenting complaint. This begins even as the patient enters for the first time, where such matters as general build, gait, colouring, tidiness, demeanour and cleanliness must be assessed. This aspect of prescribing is more relevant to the treatment of chronic diseases which are, to some degree, functionally reversible by medicinal means (such as rheumatoid arthritis, eczema, predisposition to polypus formation). This usually requires much time spent with the patient, competent use of what is termed a **repertory** (see below, *What is a repertory?*), and is less suited to busy over-the-counter (OTC) or clinical situations. It often takes a large number of consultations or assessments (at monthly intervals or less) in order to achieve satisfactory results. The 'simillimum' with regard to the general or constitutional aspects of the patient may, in some cases, be difficult to assess with ease, and the 'cure' is often achieved by a sequence of 'simillima' over the course of many months.

Although it might seem somewhat illogical to relegate the presenting complaint of a person to a position of secondary importance, and to favour those aspects of the patient which *appear to be unrelated to it*, this is not the case. If we view a particular disease as an unhealthy tree, and the basic physiology as the soil in which it grows, it follows that we may either spray the leaves of the tree directly (pathological prescribing), or treat it at the roots by modifying the soil (constitutional prescribing). Modifying the general physiology often produces more profound and lasting cures in chronic disease than is achievable with pathological prescribing alone. Ideally, a constitutional remedy should also cover the presenting complaint and its individualized symptoms. This, however, may be difficult to achieve with a single remedy. Hence many chronic diseases are treated with some combination or alternation of both constitutional and pathological remedies.

Where a chronic disease is incurable, due to severe and irreversible anatomical change (e.g. gross osteoarthritis), or where the physiology is greatly weakened by malnutrition, chronic ill-health or age, it is often better to palliate the case with pathological remedies than to offer a constitutional prescription. In the case of severe anatomical change, little good will be achieved by a constitutional prescription. In the case of a weakened physiology, much strain will be placed on it by such prescribing, which may, in itself, produce a further deterioration of the patient. In some instances an antidotal remedy may then need to be given (prescribed according to the symptomatology of the deteriorated state). This deterioration is caused by the deployment of energy to the treatment of a disease from an already depleted energy pool.

What is a repertory?

A **repertory** is quite different from a therapeutic index (see above, *How are remedies selected?*). Although a repertory may have a limited number of entries concerning conventional diagnostic categories, these do not comprise its main substance. Nor is its purpose to act as a mere substitute. The bulk of the repertory is concerned with individual objective and subjective symptoms (such as rash, pain in the face), qualifications of those symptoms (including character, modalities, laterality) and general aspects of the patient (such as thermal sensitivities, desires, aversions, food likes and dislikes, pathological predispositions, bodily conformation, colouring, and emotional status). These are classified under various headings and subheadings, termed **rubrics**. Under each rubric a number of remedies are listed, using a variety of weights of type (CAPITAL, **Bold**, *Italic*, Standard, etc.) to denote grades of importance. The idea is to select a remedy that appears to be dominantly expressed throughout a large proportion of the selected rubrics. In fact, special numerical scoring methods are taught for this purpose. One of the better ones is in Dublin Murphy's *Homeopathic Medical Repertory* (Murphy, 1993), which has a very satisfactory alphabetical arrangement. A number of computer software packages are now available (e.g. MacRepertory and Cara) which help to accelerate the process of what is termed **repertorization**, i.e. the selection of a remedy via a repertory. However, repertorization is not suited to busy OTC or clinical situations (except in the case of those more expert), and the use of a therapeutic index, under these circumstances, is more appropriate (see below, *What is a 'similior'?*).

Repertorization of thermal sensitivity

Any reader who wishes to take prescribing to a more advanced level will note that **thermal sensitivity** is often one of the best criteria with which to begin repertorization, and thus the process of selecting a simillimum. In this regard, it is appropriate to divide the universe of patients into three main classes of thermal sensitivity (cold, hot and 'ambithermal'), with respect to either their presenting complaints or their constitutional predispositions; and so similarly, the remedies used to treat them. The following example of this repertorial approach (see Box 1.1) uses 'standard' abbreviations (e.g. ARS. for *Arsenicum album*), which vary only slightly between repertories. The degree of correspondence is categorized as having three levels: FULL CAPITAL TYPE is the highest; *Italic* is intermediate; and Standard the least (after Gibson Miller).

The 'thermal' approach, as may be gathered from the entry MERC. (*Mercurius solubilis*) in Box 1.1 (last line), is applicable to both acute and chronic disease. Where the thermal sensitivity of the patient has changed, say, from hot to chilly, then a 'cold remedy' should be selected. Indeed, for the purposes of repertorization, symptoms should be gathered in groups according to their chronological development. (It thus follows that an active acute disease must be treated in preference to an underlying chronic one.) Those most recent should be repertorized first, and it is these that should guide the prescriber to the initial prescription, in conjunction, of

REMEDIES CORRESPONDING TO PERSONS OR CONDITIONS PREDOMINANTLY AGGRAVATED BY COLD ('COLD REMEDIES'):

Abrot., Acet-ac., *Acon.*, *Agar.*, *Agn.*, Alumen, *Alum.*, *Al-ph.*, *Alum-sil.*, Am-c., Apoc., *Arg-m.*, ARS. (except for headache), Ars-s-fl., Asar., *Aur.*, Aur-ars., Aur-sulph., *Bad.*, BAR-C., *Bar-m.*, *Bell.*, Benz-ac., Borax., Brom., Cadm., *Calc-ars.*, CAL-C., *Calc-fl.*, CALC-PH., *Calc-sil.*, Camph., Canth., CAPS., Carb-an., *Carb-veg.*, Carbn-sul., Card-m., *Cauloph.*, CAUST., *Cham.*, *Chel.*, CHINA., *Chin-a.*, *Cimic.*, *Cistus.*, *Cocc.*, *Coff.*, Colch., *Con.*, *Cycl.*, DULC., *Euphras.*, FERR., *Ferr-ars.*, Form., GRAPH., Guaj., *Hell.*, *Helon.*, HEP., *Hyosc.*, HYPER., *Ign.*, KALI-ARS., *Kali-bich.*, KALI-CARB., *Kali-chlor.*, Kali-phos., *Kali-sil.*, *Kalm.*, *Kreos.*, *Lac-defl.*, MAGN-CARB., MAGN-PHOS., *Mang.*, MOSCH., Mur-ac., *Natr-ars.*, *Natr-carb.*, NITRIC-AC., Nux-m., NUX-VOM., Oxal-ac., *Petrol.*, PHOS., Phos-ac., *Plb.*, *Pod.*, PSOR., PYROGEN., RAN-B., Rheum., *Rhodo.*, RHUS., RUMEX, *Ruta*, SABAD., *Sars.*, SEPIA, SIL., SPIG., *Stann.*, Staph., Stram., STRONT., *Sul-ac.*, *Therid.*, Valer., *Viol-t.*, *Zinc.*

REMEDIES CORRESPONDING TO PERSONS OR CONDITIONS PREDOMINANTLY AGGRAVATED BY HEAT ('HOT REMEDIES'):

Aesc-h., *All-c.*, *Aloe*, Ambra., APIS, ARG-NIT., *Asaf.*, *Aur-iod.*, *Aur-m.*, Bar-iod., *Bry.*, *Calad.*, *Calc-iod.*, *Calc-sul.*, *Cocc-cacti.*, Comoc., *Crocus.*, *Dros.*, Fer-iod., FLUOR-AC., *Grat.*, *Ham.*, IOD., KALI-IOD., KALI-SUL., *Lach.*, *Led.*, *Lil-t.*, *Lyc.*, NAT-MUR., NAT-SUL., Niccol., *Op.*, Picric-ac., PLAT., Ptelia, PULS., SABINA, SECALE, *Spong.*, *Sul.*, *Sul-iod.*, Thuj., Tuberc., Ustil., *Vespa.*, Viburn.

REMEDIES CORRESPONDING TO SENSITIVITY TO BOTH HOT and COLD ('AMBITHERMAL REMEDIES'):

Ant-cr. (< radiant heat, though many symptoms > by heat), Cinnabar, *Ip.*, MERC. (chronic disease < cold; acute disease < heat), Nat-carb.

Box 1.1
Repertorization of thermal sensitivity.

course, with a consideration of the general aspects of the patient (size, temperament, etc.).

One of the biggest mistakes in any selective process is to attempt to match the entirety of the symptomatic history and general characteristics of the patient against one remedy. In cases in which there are a multitude of features on which to base a prescription, failure almost inevitably results. Far better to treat such a case as being stratified, clearing each layer with some sense of planning, as any good archaeologist might do. If the first prescription works successfully, so the symptomatic picture will change to that of the next stratum, and the new picture will determine the second prescription. These, at least, are some basic principles with which to begin. With experience, however, such rules may be broken occasionally, more particularly where an underlying obstruction to cure is suspected in the form of a 'miasm' (see below, *What is a miasm?*).

The materia medica

There are numerous works on **materia medica**, in which the remedies are listed alphabetically and their properties delineated under various headings: pathological indications, susceptible typology, mind, head, eyes, nose, face, mouth, stomach, abdomen, stool, urine, male, female, respiratory, heart, back, extremities, sleep, fever, skin, modalities, relationship and comparison with other remedies, and dosage. The one to be recommended as a good basic reference work is William Boericke's *Pocket Manual of Homoeopathic Materia Medica* (Boericke, 1927).

Treated as a whole, the homeopathic materia medica has many objective and subjective signs (pathogeneses), the clinical significance of which has never or seldom been verified. These are symptoms or signs which have been caused by a drug or potentized remedy (by proving or toxicity), but, although the implication is that they might also be cured by the relevant remedy, this has not been satisfactorily confirmed. Good works of materia medica, however, emphasize which diseases and syndromes have been repeatedly cured by a particular remedy, so that we may be more certain in our choice. Indeed, there are some entries where only the curative aspect of a remedy has been observed, and not the pathogenetic.

In homeopathic prescribing, particularly at the constitutional level, much emphasis is often placed on the so-called **mentals**. So much so, that the 'mentals' are separated from the **generals**. The term 'mentals' refers to the detailed psychological status of the individual (such as weepiness, friendliness, etc.), which is often taken as a prime indication for the 'constitutional simillimum'. (However, when an acute anxiety state in relation to, say, a dental procedure is treated as an entity in itself, this is a form of *pathological*, rather than constitutional prescribing.)

Many homeopaths feel, however, that the ideal selected constitutional remedy should cover not only the mental and general aspects of the case, but also those of the presenting complaint or pathology (and, preferably, with regard also to its individual symptomatic manifestation). Therefore, where two remedies would seem to be in contest on the basis of the mental and general analysis, the one that more frequently treats the particular pathology should be selected in preference. In contrast to the generals, details concerning a particular pathology or disease (the presenting complaint), and its individualized objective and subjective symptoms, are termed the **particulars**.

What are leading symptoms?

A **leading symptom** is one that suggests the consideration of a limited number of remedies above all others – although often one of these is more commonly indicated, e.g. *excessive salivation and halitosis* with toothache: *Merc. sol.* (*Mercurius solubilis*). A leading symptom may, in fact, be a quality or modality, e.g. *throbbing* pain: *Belladonna*; toothache > *cold water in the mouth*: *Chamomilla* or *Coffea cruda*. These are leading symptoms in pathological prescribing, but the concept may also be applied to constitutional remedy selection, e.g. irritability < *especially to her nearest and dearest*: *Sepia*. Leading symptoms are also called **keynotes**.

However, when all is said and done, a remedy might be *indicated* for consideration by a leading symptom, but can only be selected as

Die in den Haus-Apotheken enthaltenen Mittel dienen in derselben Beschaffenheit zugleich zur Anwendung bei Tieren.

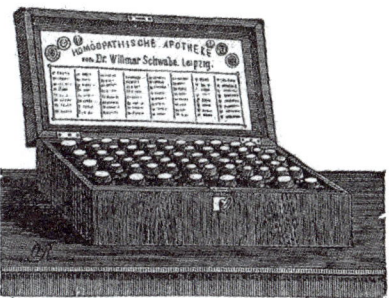

Verbesserte Haus-Apotheke mit 66 Mitteln.

6. **Apotheken in Schrankform** (Eiche oder Nussbaum) mit Flaschen von 25, 15 und 5 g.   mit 42   66   85 Mitteln
ℳ 32,50   44,—   61,—.

7. **Taschen- und Reise-Apotheken** mit Zylinder EE.
a) in Leinw.-Etuis mit 6   8   12   18   24   32   44   64 Mittl.
ℳ 2,25 3,— 4,50 6,— 7,50 — 13,50 —
b) in Leder-Etuis ℳ 4,50 — 6,50 9,— 11,— 13,50 17,50 23,50.

Brusttaschen-Etui mit 18 Mitteln ℳ 9,50.

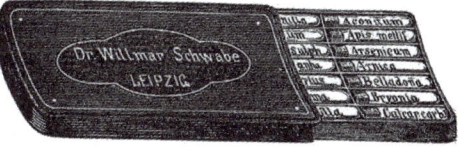

Brusttaschenetui.

Figure 1.3
German domestic remedy chest and a traveller's kit. From the pricelist of the Dr Willmar Schwabe Pharmacy, Leipzig, *c.* 1900.

appropriate if it matches in other respects. Irritability towards one's husband, in itself, is not a sufficient basis for the prescription of *Sepia*; but, where it occurs in an overworked female with bearing-down feelings in the lower abdomen (sometimes from uterine prolapse), then it becomes strongly indicated. Some talk of a **three-legged stool**, implying that much good prescribing can be achieved by finding three leading symptoms which match a particular remedy. Indeed, in the hands of the expert prescriber, it is a valid and valuable technique. For those interested in pursuing this approach, Nash's *Leaders in Homoeopathic Therapeutics* (Nash, 2002) is to be recommended for further reading.

Strange, rare or peculiar symptoms are a particular subgroup of leading symptoms, which have an enigmatic and inscrutable nature, and which lead to the consideration of particular remedies, e.g. burning sensation > *heat*: *Arsenicum album*; urgency to urinate < *putting hands in cold water*: *Kreasotum*.

Prescription by causation

Sometimes a remedy can be prescribed on the basis of the event, circumstances or disease which seemed to precipitate the presenting complaint or constitutional upset, even though this may have occurred many years previously. Frequently, the same remedy may be given as might have been possibly chosen for the precipitating disturbance itself. For example, epilepsy following concussion: *Natrum sulphuricum* (a principal remedy for concussion); not well since mechanical trauma: *Arnica* (a key remedy for mechanical trauma); not well since BCG immunization: *BCG nosode*; inflammatory arthritis from dental focal sepsis: *Hepar sulph*. (the principal remedy for chronic dental abscess).

Using a therapeutic index, repertory and materia medica

In analysing any case, the initial approach is quite different with regard to these three categories of reference work:

1. With a *therapeutic index*, we begin by selecting a conventional category of disease/syndrome. This is the easiest method in busy OTC and clinical situations.
2. With a *repertory*, we usually begin by selecting a number of general and mental characteristics, or objective and subjective symptoms.
3. With a *materia medica*, we begin by selecting particular remedies for consideration, based on personal clinical experience, on the suggestions of a therapeutic index, or on the results of repertorization. A standard and comprehensive work of materia medica is thus the ultimate source of information.

What is a miasm?

The term **miasm** (plural: miasms/miasmata) or, more correctly, **chronic miasm**, is applied to various diagnostic entities in homeopathy:

1. A familial genetic trait (such as thyroid disease).
2. An inherited Lamarckian disease trait stemming from ancestral infection (e.g the tuberculous miasm from ancestral TB, which may lead to bronchitic tendencies in the descendants).
3. The prolonged aftermath of an infection or immunization (e.g. postviral syndrome, epilepsy following measles immunization, a tuberculous miasm following TB in the individual himself).
4. The prolonged aftermath of drug or chemical toxicity when the causative agent is no longer present in the body.

Remedies such as *Bacillinum* (one of several TB nosodes) and *Medorrhinum* (gonococcal nosode) are essentially anti-miasmatic, and are generally given infrequently for the treatment of chronic disease. However, *Medorrhinum* is also an *acute* remedy in its own right for the treatment of acute otitis media and the prevention of barotauma.

Where there have been problems in finding an appropriate remedy via repertory or materia medica, the existence of an underlying miasm may be suspected. Such a conclusion, however, depends on the level of skill of the practitioner (for failure to find the remedy can result merely from inexperience), and the elimination of nutritional, psychological, sociological and patho-anatomical obstructions to treatment. For the genuine miasm, special anti-miasmatic remedies, such as those given above, may be required. Otherwise, the case is sometimes 'cleared' with a few doses of high potency *Sulphur*. Where it is fairly obvious that a non-inherited miasm has been caused by a particular infective episode in the history of the patient himself (e.g. glandular fever, whooping cough), then a nosode made from the offending micro-organism is often administered. A similar approach can be adopted with post-immunization syndromes. Where it is believed that a certain drug has lead to the miasm, then a remedy made from that drug may be given.

The classically described chronic miasmata of homeopathy are:

- psora (suppressed itch disease – usually scabies)
- syphilis (from the disease of the same name)
- sycosis (fig-wart disease – from a mixture of gonorrhoea *and* wart virus).

These entities are actually more of historic and academic interest, though they do also have some limited clinical usefulness, even these days (Speight, 1991). They are perhaps best regarded as hereditary clinical syndromes, though not necessarily of infective origin, as once thought.

What is 'Hering's Law'?

Constantine Hering (1800–80) was one of Hahnemann's more important pupils. **Hering's Law**, which first appeared in a preface to Hempel's translation of Hahnemann's *Chronic Diseases*, Volume 1 (Hahnemann, 1845), gives us the means of assessing the correct progression of curative (constitutional) treatment of a *chronic* disease:

Cure occurs from above downwards, from within outwards, and in reverse chronological order.

Put simply, this means that the cure is proceeding successfully when the upper bodily symptoms clear before the lower, when more important organs (e.g. the lungs) improve before those of lesser fundamental importance (e.g. the skin), and when old symptoms return briefly, the most recent appearing first. Although not all these points may be observed in any particular case, the occurrence of inverse responses is regarded as an indication of incorrect therapy. Hence, where the symptoms clear from below upwards, or from the skin to the lungs, or in chronological order of their development, then the treatment is unsatisfactory and not curative.

One thing that is not uncommon in the successful treatment of a chronic disease is the occurrence of a transient skin rash, even in a patient with no history of skin disorder. This is termed **externalization**, and is usually regarded as a strong indication that the treatment is progressing satisfactorily. Nevertheless, it also indicates that the intensity of the therapy should be reduced (by giving a lower potency, less frequent repetition, or a respite from treatment).

Potencies and frequency of repetition

For the beginner, the best thing to do initially with regard to potency and repetition of dose is to follow the directives of a therapeutic index as closely as possible. Always stop the prescription if apparent proving (see above, *More about cause and cure*) or **aggravation** occurs, and avoid giving anything other than low potencies (i.e. 6c–9c) in pregnancy. **Aggravation** is where the remedy appears to worsen the existing symptoms, the causes of which are discussed further in Chapter 3 (see also Chapter 4, *Adverse effects of potentized remedies*). Also carefully note my comments on Hering's Law (see above, *What is 'Hering's Law'?*).

Although the usual advice is to discontinue any treatment for an *acute* illness as soon as the patient is fully recovered, it is better, in my own experience, to continue it for a further 24–48 hours, in order to prevent relapse – except in ultra-acute cases, such as collapse or acute epistaxis (nosebleed). Whilst, at least in theory, clinical proving might result from this prolongation of therapy, in actual practice this is extremely rare, and the advantages of such prolongation outweigh the disadvantages.

What is a 'similior'?

The pathological simillimum may be regarded as a match against symptoms/signs of the first degree. We might call a poor match one of the third degree, and this would be of limited clinical use. Even worse would be a *mismatch* of the fourth degree, produced by 'sticking a pin' in a list of remedies. As you will now appreciate, in actual practice the selection of the simillimum in the *true* sense of the word (i.e. 'the *most* similar') may be extremely difficult for the newcomer. Fortunately, nature gives us much leeway and allows us to give remedies of the second degree, which we may term **similiores** (Latin: 'those *more* similar'). The selection of a **similior** (my own word, I might add) often yields perfectly satisfactory clinical results, despite the relative inexactitude of the symptom/sign matching process.

A *therapeutic index* will help you find at least a similior, if not the simillimum itself, with comparative ease. Therapeutic indexes use a variety of methods to speed up the remedy selection process, the main ones being:

- a statistical approach based on clinical experience – the remedy most likely to cure the majority of cases is listed first (and sometimes solely). Where the disease to be treated is of a contagious or infectious nature, this remedy is termed the **genus epidemicus**.
- including symptomatic or constitutional information, which must be taken into account for the remedy to be considered a possible pathological simillimum or similior.
- suggesting a complex or combination remedy (see Chapter 4, *Complex prescriptions*), at least one component of which is

likely to be a similior (or even the pathological simillimum). In some instances, two or more remedies in the complex may even work together to produce a more desirable outcome than might have been achieved by the use of one alone. Such remedies may be said to be 'complementary', although this term has traditionally been applied to sequential, rather than complex, prescriptions. Indeed, the index may suggest particular sequences or alternations of different remedies (rather than complexes), which are held in high regard therapeutically.

Homeopathic remedies are made from a wide variety of 'substances' – animal, vegetable, mineral (natural or synthetic), gaseous, bacterial, viral, and electromagnetic – and it is not unusual for a specialist pharmacy to stock over 3000 varieties, in different therapeutic strengths. In fact, with increasing public and professional demand for them, together with positive clinical validation, they are now to be considered as major pharmaceutical products which are here to stay.

2 Thinking about how remedies are made

Introduction

Most of the methods used in modern homeopathic pharmaceutical practice derive directly from the work of Samuel Hahnemann MD (see Figure 2.2) (1755–1843) in the late eighteenth and early nineteenth centuries, as published in various editions of his *Organon* (see Figure 2.1) and elsewhere (e.g. Hahnemann, 1845). It will come as no surprise that they have undergone some modification since then. This has been driven principally by the need for greater production in the face of increasing international demand from both practitioners and public alike. Nevertheless, the fundamental techniques of homeopathic pharmaceutics still remain essentially the same. What we have added are a greater efficiency through mechanization, a vastly increased armamentarium of remedies, a few new methods of preparation, and perhaps a better insight into their physicochemical nature. Some things have been lamentably lost, others laudably gained. Notwithstanding these issues, homeopathic pharmaceutics is a science and art which involves several ingenious techniques quite different from those of its allopathic (conventional) and botanic (herbal) counterparts. Indeed, it is something of infinite fascination to those who have been fortunate enough to practise it.

Pharmaceutical objectives

It is true that homeopathy sometimes uses raw or simply diluted tinctures in therapy internally or externally, thus causing confusion with herbalism. But this usage is restricted, and not indicative of what homeopathic pharmacy is really about. It was found, early in the history of homeopathy, that drugs administered on the basis of the **Similia Principle** (see Chapter 1, *Introduction*) could be given effectively in much smaller doses than those commonly used in allopathic medicine of the same era.

Although small by allopathic standards of the time, the original dosages employed in the homeopathic manner were still of significant size, e.g. *Opium* 31mg. However, it was subsequently discovered that, provided drugs were prepared in particular ways and applied according to the Similia Principle, these doses could be reduced even further. Indeed, they could be given in infinitesimal doses, not only without loss of efficacy, but often with gain in therapeutic strength, and lack of the initial aggravations of disease symptomatology that often followed their use in significant material quantity. Furthermore, it was found that substances which were pharmacologically inert in the raw state, such as quartz and graphite, would develop medicinal properties when subjected to the procedures of homeopathic pharmacy. The potential clinical indications of such inert substances could only be determined by administering them to sensitive persons in the properly prepared form, and recording their subjective and objective symptomatic effects. In that way, it was possible to use them clinically in accordance with the Similia Principle.

The particular collection of methods used to prepare substances homeopathically is termed **potentization** or **dynamization**. Conventional potentization involves serial dilution, together with serial energization – that is to say, the delivery of mechanical energy after each stage of dilution. There are two types of conventional potentization:

1. *Liquid phase potentization*, using ethanol–water as the diluent, and succussion (vigorous agitation) or fluxion (jetting) as the means of mechanical energization.
2. *Solid phase potentization*, using lactose as the diluent, and trituration (vigorous grinding) to supply mechanical energy.

The primary objectives of potentization may be defined as follows:

1. To reduce the toxicity of a substance (e.g. mercury, arsenic). This is achieved by serial dilution alone.
2. To transfer the molecular or ionic geometry of a substance to the **molecular memory** of the diluent (**imprinting**), and to progressively intensify such information (**intensification**). In this respect, note the following two points:
    i. Whereas serial dilution gradually diminishes the presence of the 'original substance', this is replaced by molecules of diluent which have been imprinted with its molecular or

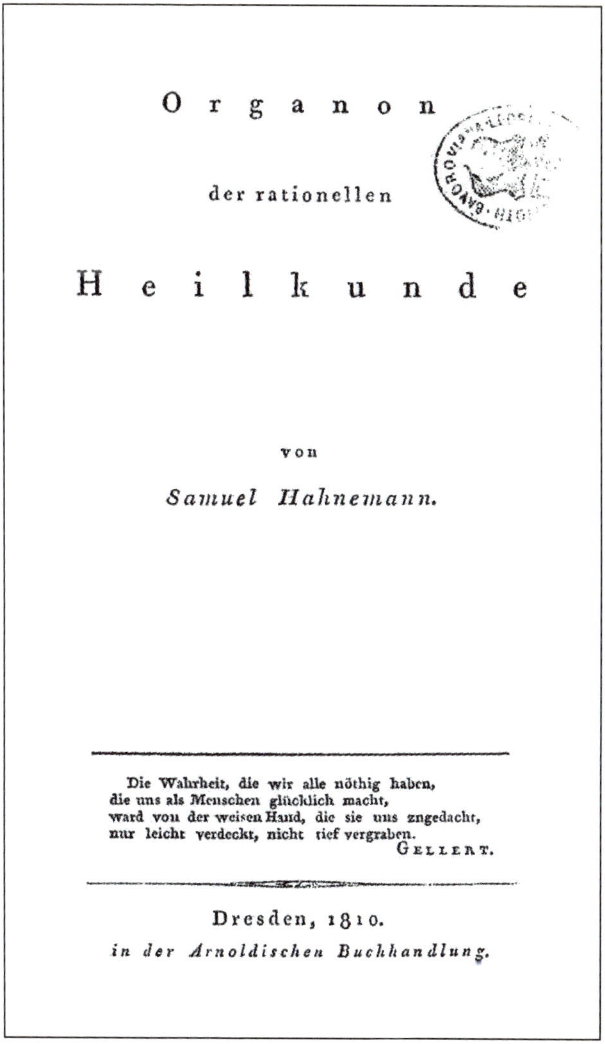

Organon

der rationellen

Heilkunde

von

Samuel Hahnemann.

Die Wahrheit, die wir alle nöthig haben,
die uns als Menschen glücklich macht,
ward von der weisen Hand, die sie uns zugedacht,
nur leicht verdeckt, nicht tief vergraben.
GELLERT.

Dresden, 1810.
in der Arnoldischen Buchhandlung.

Figure 2.1
Title page of the first edition of Hahnemann's *Organon*, 1810 (Dresden, Arnold). The first comprehensive textbook of homeopathy.

ionic **imagery**. Thus, as serial dilution continues, these imprinted molecules become of great importance in the transfer of such information to new molecules of diluent introduced into the preparatory vessel.
   ii. Imprinting and intensification are sometimes referred to conjointly by the term 'potentization', irrespective of the means by which they are produced (i.e. conventionally or otherwise).
3. To develop the medicinal properties of a substance which is initially pharmacologically inert (e.g. flint, which becomes the remedy *Silicea/Silica*).
4. To remove old 'memories' from the diluent – that is to say, to 'overwrite' them with new information. This is only possible where such memories are of weak intensity, which is usually the case with any diluent which has not been previously subjected to pharmaceutical potentization.

Scales of serial dilution

For those unfamiliar with our numerical definitions of dilution, it must be explained, by way of example, that a dilution of 1 in 100 in homeopathic pharmacy may mean any of the following, according to the mode of preparation, and when it arose historically:

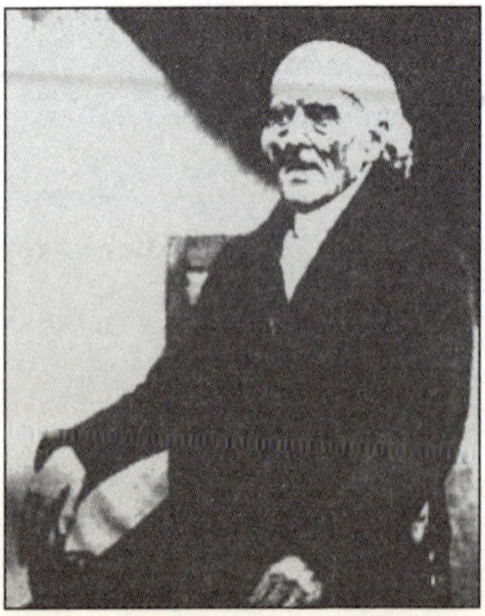

Figure 2.2
Samuel Hahnemann. From a daguerrotype taken 30 September 1841 in Paris.

- 1 drop in 100 drops (about 4.5ml)
- 1 grain (62 or 65mg) in 100 drops
- 1g in 100ml (1dl)
- 1 grain in 100 minims (1 minim = 0.0592ml)
- 1 grain in 100 grains
- 1g in 100g.

The three scales of serial dilution, given in order of historical development, are as follows (although the first and third are more popular than the second).

1. The **centesimal** scale: serial dilutions of 1 in 100. Invented by Hahnemann. Abbreviations: c, cH, CH, H, or nothing! Thus, the sixth centesimal dilution (1 in 10^{12}), or **potency**, may be labelled: 6c, 6cH, 6CH, 6H, or 6. Generally 6c is the version used in the UK and USA. Once we get to a potency of 1000c – where serial dilution and energization have been carried out 1000 times – the abbreviation changes to M or, better still, 1M. Hence: 10M = 10 000c, 50M = 50 000c, and CM = 100 000c. After CM, little or no increase in therapeutic activity can be expected.
2. The **fifty millesimal** scale: serial dilutions of 1 in 50 000 (or thereabouts), though the first potency of the scale (LM1) is traditionally prepared from the 3c potency of an original substance. This is the second scale invented by Hahnemann, but the manuscript describing it was lost until the early twentieth century. By this time, the centesimal and decimal (see below) scales had become firmly ensconced, and it is only relatively recently that interest in the fifty millesimal has become significant. Abbreviations: LM or Q. So, LM1, LM2 or Q1, Q2, right up to LM30 or Q30.
3. The **decimal** scale: serial dilutions of 1 in 10. Developed after Hahnemann's death by his followers. Abbreviations: D (sometimes DH), x. Thus, D12 = 12x. D is favoured more in continental Europe, especially in Central Europe (where the decimal scale itself is more popular), and will be used in this book for its clarity. In the UK, requests for decimal potencies higher than 30x (D30) are rare.

A 6c, therefore, has undergone the same degree of dilution as a D12 'potency', i.e. 1 in 10^{12}. However, the 6c has experienced only 6 episodes of serial energization, whereas the D12 has experienced 12. From this alone it should be concluded that their physical properties are likely to differ. From the practical point of view, D- and c-scale preparations of the same *numerical* value (e.g. D6 and 6c), though *not* those of the same level of dilution, may be regarded as therapeutically similar up to a value of about 30 (for further discussion, see below, *Classical energization: succussion*). Direct comparisons of LM potencies with c and D potencies are imprecise, but it may be said that LM1 produces therapeutic effects rather like those of a 30c/D30, and LM2 produces therapeutic effects rather like those of a 200c. There are, however, other differences in terms of adverse patient reaction (see below, *Manufacture of LMs*).

Technically, to prepare the first centesimal potency (1c) of a mother tincture, first of all 1 drop should be added to 99 drops of ethanol–water (but, as we shall see later, this is not always the case – see below, *Impurities*). The vial is then tightly stoppered with an unbleached cork, succussion performed (see below, *Classical energization: succussion*), and the vial labelled 1c. Thereafter, 1 drop of the succussed 'liquid potency' is transferred to a new vial containing 99 drops of ethanol–water, and a new cork inserted. This is then succussed to produce the 2c potency (cumulative dilution: 1 in 10^4), which is so labelled. One drop of this is then transferred to another new vial containing 99 drops of diluent, a new cork procured, and succussion again carried out to yield the 3c potency (cumulative dilution: 1 in 10^6). And so on. Decimal scale liquid phase potentization is similar in principle, but 1 drop is added to 9 of diluent. Also, as Hahnemann (1845) states: 'Vials that have contained one medicine ought never to be used for any other, even if they should have been previously rinsed ever so much' (although, as we shall discuss later, they may be recycled by applying heat – see below, *Erasure of imprinting*)

Electromagnetic remedies (see below, *Electromagnetic potentization*) are handled similarly, as are liquid preparations made from animal, bacterial or viral materials. There are also a number of salts (e.g. copper sulphate – *Cuprum sulphuricum*) and other substances which, being soluble in distilled water, may be subjected to liquid phase potentization in the same way as mother tinctures, and without the necessity for prior serial trituration. In the second half of the nineteenth century and first half of the twentieth, 10 grains (650mg) of such a substance would have been dissolved in sufficient water to raise the volume to 1000 or 100 minims (59.2 or 5.92ml) accordingly, to yield dilutions of 1 in 100 (centesimal) and 1 in 10 (decimal) respectively; thereafter producing the first potency by succussion (1c and D1). These days, however, many will prefer to use 1g in 100ml or 1g in 10ml, according to scale. For further stages of potentization of these materials, the alcohol content of the diluent is gradually increased.

In contrast with the conventional method of serial dilution, that of **Korsakov**, developed in 1829, has the advantage of using only a single preparatory vial. After succussion, the contents of the vial are sucked or tipped out, leaving the equivalent of 1 drop adherent to its inner surface. To this, 99 drops of diluent are added, and the process repeated. The resultant potencies are sometimes denoted by the suffix K or cK, e.g. 6cK. The most important current application of the Korsakovian method is in mechanical devices used to produce very high potencies (see below, *Fluxion*).

The following points should be noted concerning 'the drop' as a dispensing measurement:

1. Drops will vary in size according to the nature and concentration of their solute and, more importantly, their alcohol content. The higher the concentration of alcohol, the smaller the drop.
2. Drops also vary according to the manner in which they are dispensed. Often, in the case of a mother tincture or liquid potency, the vial is tipped and its cork is carefully loosened to allow 1 drop to fall. The more tapered the cork, the smaller the drop. Glass pipettes and capillary tubes may be used to better advantage, but these too will deliver varying sizes of drops, according to their dimensions (see Figure 2.3). Beyond that, a glass device which has been used for one liquid potency must not be used for another. It must,

therefore, be kept for dispensing that item alone, or else disposed of or recycled with heat treatment (see below, *Erasure of imprinting*).

3. In terms of traditional pharmacy, a 'standard drop' should be 1 minim, or 0.0592ml, at 16.7°C (for the word 'minim' really means a 'dispensable minimum of liquid', i.e. a 'drop'). This is a measurement based on pure water. Since, however, homeopaths mainly deal with alcohol–water, we must regard a 'standard homeopathic drop' as something smaller. In this respect, 0.045ml is more realistic. Even so, in actual practice, there may be as much as 15% deviation on either side of this figure, for the reasons just given. Nevertheless, and perhaps surprisingly, the effect of such variability on the qualities of the remedy so produced is fairly minimal.

4. It will thus be apparent that numerical statements concerning homeopathic dilutions involving drops (e.g. 1 in 100) are really approximations. Hahnemann himself, being aware of this fact, states with regard to centesimal serial dilutions: 'Of this solution you again take one drop, and mix it with 99 or 100 drops of pure alcohol' (Hahnemann, 1845).

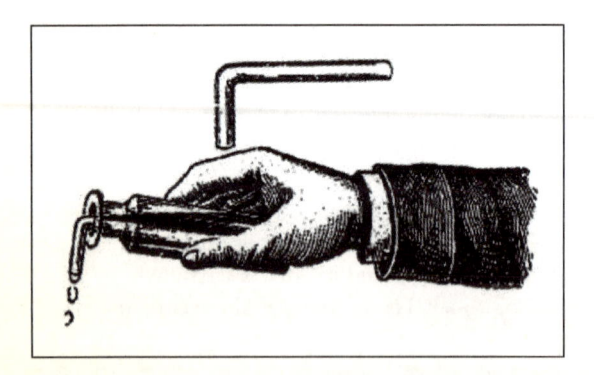

Figure 2.3
Capillary tube for regulating drops. From the pricelist of the Dr Willmar Schwabe Pharmacy, Leipzig, *c.* 1900.

5. It is more convenient to dispense larger quantities of drops in millilitres. For example, 4.5ml may be taken to be more or less equal to 99 or 100 drops, although here again different pharmacies may hold different opinions.

Furthermore, and by way of example, when we announce that a 30c potency represents a dilution of 1 in 10^{60} (which, in terms of concentration, is 10^{-60}), such a numerical statement of cumulative dilution is only notional since, at this level of potentization, there is very little probability that any molecules or ions of the original substance remain. Whilst we have traditionally assumed that this is essentially the case with all potencies above 12c or D24, recent work has suggested that the concentration of such molecules or ions tends to exceed that predicted by the level of dilution and, thus, that they may persist to some minor, though significant, degree beyond 'Avogadro's point' (Samal and Geckeler, 2001) − not that anyone should get too excited, since this does not explain the therapeutic effects of the higher potencies.

The matter of serial dilution as it applies to the trituration of substances with lactose is considered later in some detail (see below, *Classical energization: trituration*).

Manufacture of LMs

It is believed that **LM potencies** are less prone to produce aggravation of existing symptoms than the c and D scales. The matter of aggravation and its causes is discussed in more detail in Chapter 3.

The mode of preparation of LM potencies is somewhat more complicated than that described for c- and D-scale preparations, and was Hahnemann's last pharmaceutical bequest to posterity. The dilutions involved are not at all straightforward:

1. Classically, the original substance, whether soluble or insoluble in alcohol–water, is serially triturated with lactose to the 3c level.
2. Following Hahnemann's instructions precisely, 1 Nuremberg grain (62mg) of the 3c potency is dissolved in 400 drops

of distilled water plus 100 drops of 90% alcohol, i.e. in 500 drops in total, or 22.5ml.
Simple dilution, i.e. without succussion: 1 grain of triturated material in 500 drops.

3. One drop of this solution is placed in another vial with 100 drops of 95% alcohol (total: 101 drops), and this is corked and succussed 100 times (see below, *Classical energization: succussion*).
Dilution: 1 grain of triturated material in 50 500 drops.

4. A few drops of this dilution are used to saturate fine sugar globules or granules (about the size of poppy seeds – see Chapter 4: Table 4.1) contained in a porcelain, glass or silver thimble with a small drainage hole at its base to allow any surplus to exit. (Each globule, weighing 1/100th of a Nuremberg grain, absorbs a little *less* than 1/500th of 1 drop.) Following saturation, they are allowed to dry superficially on filter paper. These are then stored and labelled 'LM1'.
Dilution: 1 grain of triturated material in 50 500 drops.

5. One globule or granule (= <1/500th of 1 drop) of LM1 is then used to prepare the next potency, by first dissolving it in 1 drop of distilled water in a new vial, to which are added 100 drops of 95% alcohol (total: 101 drops). A new cork is procured, and the vial is succussed 100 times. Fresh globules of the same size are then saturated with this liquid in a new thimble. These are allowed to dry, and labelled 'LM2'.
Dilution: <1 drop of LM1 in 50 500 drops = >[1 in 50 500]; or <1 grain of triturated material in $(50\,500)^2$ drops = $>[1 \text{ in } (50\,500)^2]$.

6. The procedure is repeated up to LM30.
Dilution: <1 drop of LM1 in $(50\,500)^{29}$ drops = $>[1 \text{ in } (50\,500)^{29}]$; or <1 grain of triturated material in $[50\,500]^{30}$ drops = $>[1 \text{ in } (50\,500)^{30}]$.

Nowadays, not all pharmacies prepare their LM potencies in precisely the way outlined above. Variations include the following:

- Stage 2 may be carried out using 60mg, or even only 50mg, of the 3c trituration.
- In Stage 2, some pharmacies prefer to use 1 drop of the 3c liquid phase potency of all substances soluble in alcohol–water, such as mother tinctures or various salts. Theoretically, this produces variations in the properties of the remedy, but only to a minor degree.
- In Stage 2, some pharmacies use the mother tincture directly, rather than its 3c liquid potency. This is significantly incorrect.

Mother tinctures

About 65% of all homeopathic remedies are derived from plants (Kayne, 1997). Specialist manufacturers convert them mainly into mother tinctures (alcoholic extracts), according to the directions of the various modern homeopathic pharmacopoeiae (British, German, French, American, European, Indian, Brazilian). There are three basic traditional methods for producing the mother tinctures of vegetable substances (BHP, 1882):

1. By alcoholic *percolation*, using an apparatus called a 'percolator' (see Figure 2.4). This process is used in all cases of dry plants, roots, seeds, etc., and in the case of fresh plants which are not subjected to the following two procedures. Dry material is first reduced to a moderately fine powder in a mortar; fresh plant material is minced.
2. By *maceration* (lengthy soaking) in alcohol, then *percolation*. This process is merely a modification of the former, and is applicable to fresh vegetable substances which have much mucilaginous or viscid juice, and hence will not allow alcohol to percolate readily. The material is first reduced to a pulp.
3. By *maceration* in alcohol. This process is preferable in the case of some gums, resins, etc., which are almost entirely soluble in alcohol. The material is first either reduced to a coarse powder, or cut into small pieces. Rather similarly,

phosphorus, though not a vegetable substance, will produce a saturated solution in absolute (not less than 99% wt/wt) alcohol, containing about 2mg/ml. Iodine (*Iodum*), another non-vegetable material, is soluble in rectified spirit (95% alcohol vol./vol.).

An important aspect of the manufacture of vegetable mother tinctures is the adjustment of the strength and volume of alcohol used according to the water content of the plant material, this being assessed by weighing a sample before and after drying at a temperature between 60°C and 105°C, depending on its nature. In this manner, the concentration of alcohol can be maintained at a level sufficient to guarantee its extractive and preservative properties. It is traditional to aim for a finished product which contains all the soluble matter of 1 part by weight of the *dry* plant in 10 parts by volume of the tincture (formerly 1 grain in 10 minims, and currently 1g in 10ml).

Nevertheless, there is a decided lack of uniformity between pharmacies, both in terms of the parts of the plants procured, and the way in which they are processed. The length of time recommended for maceration, for example, is very variable. To this must be added the problem of medicinal plants being prone to chemical differences according to soil, general climate and level of atmospheric pollution. Despite the availability of various sophisticated tests (e.g. NMR spectroscopy), some of which seem to be in-house secrets, standardization of mother tinctures (both between and within pharmacies) is still far from satisfactory, leading to some variation in the properties of remedies derived from them. There may be variations not only between the products of different manufacturers, but also between different batches from one and the same source. Assay of the 'principal active ingredient' – the orthodox approach – whilst often relatively straightforward, is too limited for homeopathic purposes, since we really need to know the relative concentrations of all the plant's major constituents (see below, *Impurities*). Nevertheless, provided that mother tinctures are obtained from reputable companies, such variations generally appear to be of minor clinical importance.

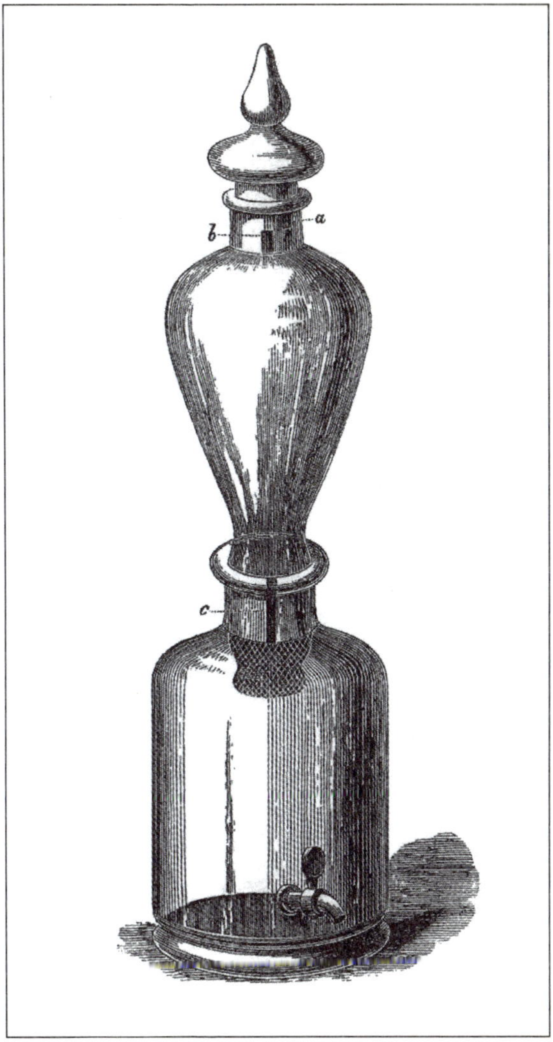

Figure 2.4
York Glass Company's percolator. For the production of mother tinctures.
London, *British Homoeopathic Pharmacopoeia*, 1882.

The symbol for mother tincture is Φ (Greek phi). This is the closest standard typographical equivalent to an ancient spagyric sigil, meaning 'spirit', 'essence' or 'essential principle'. Indeed, the plural form 'spirits' for strong alcohol is derived from this notion. It is also interesting to observe that the alcohol–water used to extract the plant is traditionally known as the *menstruum* since, to the chemists of antiquity, the process of extraction was highly feminine – a form of giving birth to the spirit of the plant. An alternative abbreviation for 'mother tincture' is MT (or TM in French-speaking countries).

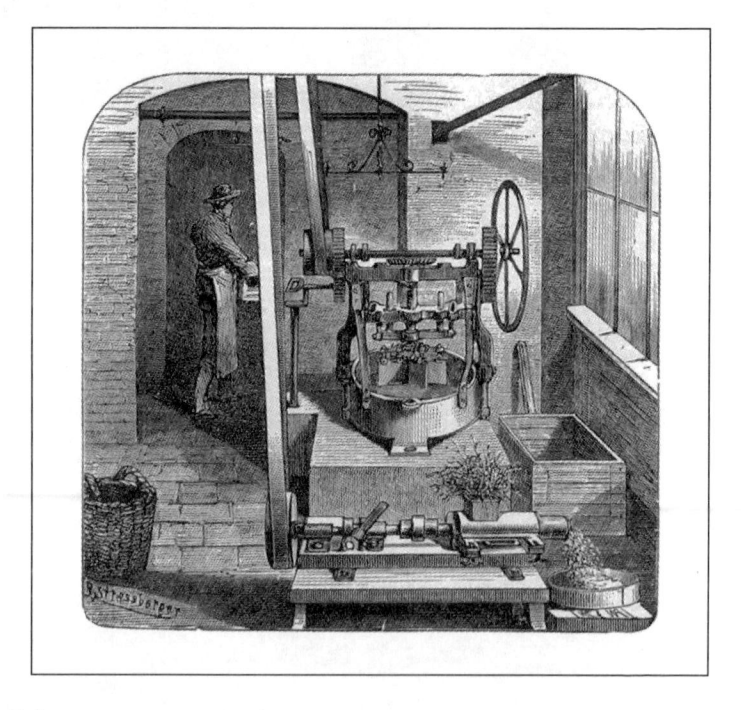

Figure 2.5
Herb and plant press. German illustration, *c.* 1920. The plant material is first minced in the device in the foreground. Expressing the sap (and then preserving it in alcohol as required) is consistent with Hahnemann's departure from the use of traditional mother tinctures from about 1835.

Mother tinctures are subjected to liquid phase potentization with ethanol water. This, indeed, is the usual way in which plant material is currently processed. Hahnemann himself abandoned the use of mother tinctures from about 1835 until the time of his death, favouring instead either freshly squeezed sap preserved in alcohol (see Figure 2.5), or pulverized dried preparations. These were then triturated with lactose up to 3c (dilution: 1 in 10^6). Thereafter the 3c was dissolved in water, alcohol added, and potentization continued in the liquid phase (see below, *Classical energization: succussion*). For the moment, however, it should be noted that all substances at a dilution of 1 in 10^6 (= 3c or D6) will go into solution or colloidal suspension in alcohol–water, irrespective of their initial state of solubility.

Diluents

Apart from the more usual meaning of the term 'diluent', in homeopathy there is another implication. This arises from the fact that the diluent is also regarded as a recording or imprinting medium for geometric information concerning the molecules and ions of the original substance from which the remedy is prepared.

The standard diluents (see Figure 2.6) are ethanol, water and lactose – or, more precisely, hydrated α-lactose. Now, if these

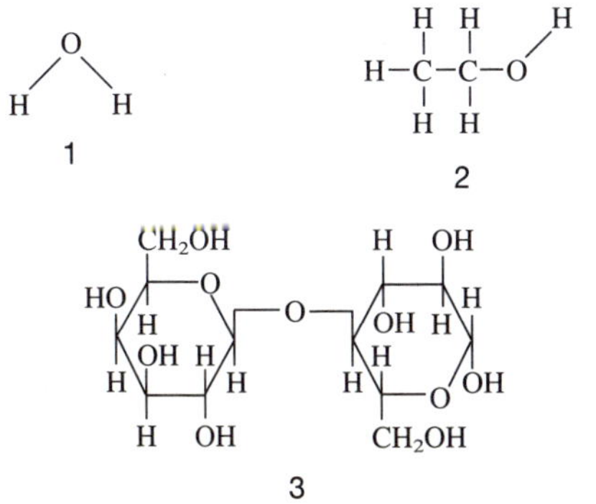

Figure 2.6
The three standard diluents of homeopathic pharmacy. **1**: Water. **2**: Ethanol. **3**: Lactose, $C_{12}H_{22}O_{11}$, H_2O (its water of crystallization is not illustrated). Lactose is a disaccharide composed of one molecule of glucose linked to one of galactose.

substances could be imprinted on themselves, bearing in mind that the presence of the diluent dominates at every stage of serial dilution, then all our remedies would convey their imprint, rather than that of any other. We may assume, therefore, that such substances are 'excluded' from the imprinting process. Besides this, a diluent must, of course, be non-toxic in the dosages normally given.

It may be proposed that, as far as imprinting is concerned, non-ionized molecules and ions are either imprinted or excluded separately, which is thus the way they should be properly considered. Therefore, Na^+Cl^- is registered as Na^+ and Cl^-, rather than NaCl. However, the matter of 'exclusion' is more complex. For any non-ionized molecule or ion to exhibit molecular memory, yet not convey its own imprint to other non-ionized molecules or ions (i.e. to be excluded), it is possible to deduce that it must conform to *all* of the chemical criteria below (this being a more extensive list than I have hitherto given):

1. It must be composed of either of the following, and of no other element:
   a. C, H and O atoms.
   b. H and O atoms.
2. It must have at least one –OH (hydroxyl) group.
3. It must have at least one H atom uninvolved in the formation of an –OH group.
4. It must have no free $>C=O$ (carbonyl) groups.
5. It must have no benzene rings.
6. It must not contain unsaturated carbon pairs $>C=C<$.

This definition does, in fact, cover quite a few substances, including: water, certain alcohols (e.g. ethanol, methanol), polysaccharides (e.g. cellulose and starch – but not chitin, which contains nitrogen and carbonyl groups), and sucrose. Additionally, lactose, glucose, and fructose, when procured pharmaceutically in solid form, exhibit cyclic structures which conform to the above criteria. In practice, this means that lactose is capable of bearing the imprints of other molecules and ions during trituration, yet offers no imprint of itself. Glucose and fructose would behave similarly, were they

Thinking about how remedies are made 41

to be present (as they might be in the case of certain desiccated original substances, e.g. dried plant sap or fruit). However, in solution, all these sugars alternate between different cyclic isomers, with intermediate open chain forms. The open chain isomers, unlike the cyclic, display free carbonyl groups (see Figure 2.7). This means, in effect, that their soluble forms cannot act as agents of molecular memory. Indeed, it might be further thought that this exhibition of free carbonyl groups would lead to their own imprinting on alcohol and water – for molecules or ions which do not comply with the above criteria usually have this propensity. Nevertheless, at any one time there is only a very small amount of the open chain form present, so this can only happen to the most minor degree (see below, *Impurities*). For example, the proportion of open chain fructose in total fructose is 0.006–0.03%. Furthermore, when a 3c trituration is dissolved in water or alcohol–water (see above, *Mother tinctures*), then the lactose molecules immediately lose any imprint on molecular memory that they have gained via this dry process, this information being conveyed almost instantly to the molecules of the liquid diluent.

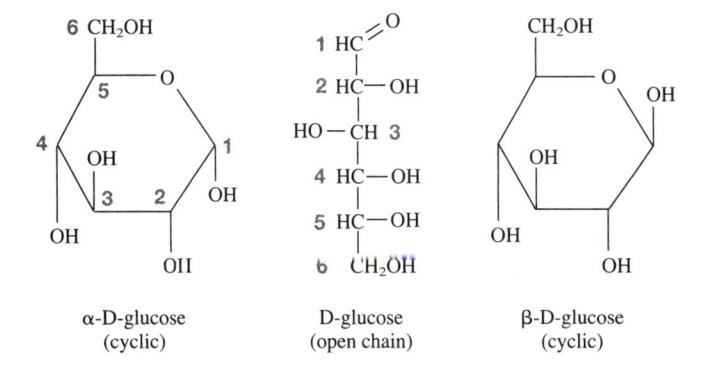

Figure 2.7
Glucose isomers. The open chain form has a free carbonyl group.

Water, as is well known, can ionize to H_3O^+ and OH^-. A brief look again at our six criteria (see page 40) will show that the H_3O^+ ion complies with them, whilst the OH^- does not. However, the ionization of water is so weak that the small amount of OH^- ions generated essentially make no imprint on molecular memory. The reason for this will become apparent, when we come to consider the matter of impurities (see below, *Impurities*).

Obviously, some of the substances that satisfy our six criteria would be totally unsuitable as diluents in homeopathy. Methanol, for example, is reasonably toxic, and cellulose is not as workable as lactose. However, the important thing to note is that they may be present in the original substance, yet do not contribute their imprint to the resultant remedy.

Impurities

Impurities may be found in the substance to be subjected to potentization or in the diluent. Some arise from atmospheric contamination (e.g. dust, fungal spores), others are leached from the inner surfaces of vials (e.g. Na^+), and particles of cork become detached from stoppers. In the case of trituration, material (e.g. silica) is abraded from both mortar and pestle. Atmospheric gases are always present in solution in liquid phase preparations, and in the form of bubbles, as a result of succussion. Such impurities seem to have little influence on the clinical properties of the potentized remedy. How can this be so?

First of all, it should be said that the imprinting of information on a diluent is most likely a 'mural phenomenon'. That is to say, it occurs between those relatively stable molecules which are situated in close apposition to the inner surface of the wall of the preparatory vessel. During succussion, the presence of large numbers of bubbles of atmospheric gases in the bulk of the solution will make no difference, since they have little or no access to this 'marginal zone' unless injected under pressure (see below, *Bubbling and prepotentization*). Particles of dust and fragments of cork behave similarly. Indeed, in the case of liquid phase potentization, the influence of all insoluble entities may be disposed of by means of this concept. Trituration, however, is a different matter, for whilst small pockets of gas are effectively 'squeezed out' of the marginal zone, and thus excluded from potentization at a relatively early stage, dust particles, lactose contaminants and abraded material are not denied such access. So, we are still left with this problem, plus that of soluble impurities in the liquid phase. In order to resolve these, we must look into the influence on imprinting of relative concentration in the marginal zone.

It can be suggested theoretically and approximately that, for the first stage of serial dilution and energization, the maximum degree Γ to which the geometry of any such molecule or ion can be imprinted on the diluent is equal to the square of its relative concentration Ψ, i.e. $\Gamma = \Psi^2$ (Lessell, 2002). However, Γ is more conveniently expressed as a percentage $\Gamma\%$, so that $\Gamma\% = 100\Psi^2$. The relative concentration Ψ_m of an imprintable molecule or ion M is calculated by dividing its absolute concentration A_m, expressed in terms of weight per unit volume, by the sum ΣA of the absolute concentrations of all the imprintable molecules and ions which are present, i.e. $\Psi_m = A_m/\Sigma A$. This applies to both solid and liquid phase methods, and equally to both true solutes and substances in colloidal suspension.

Example 1

Let us consider two hypothetical molecules, X and Y, where $A_x = 8g/dl$, $A_y = 2g/dl$, and $A_x + A_y = \Sigma A = 10g/dl$. Thus $\Psi_x = A_x/\Sigma A = 8/10 = 0.8$, and $\Psi_y = A_y/\Sigma A = 2/10 = 0.2$. On the basis of Ψ alone, it might be assumed that the relative influence of these two molecules or ions on molecular memory would be 4:1, since $\Psi_x/\Psi_y = 0.8/0.2 = 4$. However, when we apply $\Gamma\% = 100\Psi^2$, we obtain the following results:

1. $[\Gamma\%]_x = 100(0.8)^2 = 64\%$
2. $[\Gamma\%]_y = 100(0.2)^2 = 4\%$
3. $[\Gamma\%]_x / [\Gamma\%]_y = 64/4 = 16$

From these equations it can be seen that the influence of molecule X on the molecular memory of the diluent, though less than the

80% that might have been anticipated, is now 16 times that of Y. This is why impurities, the relative concentrations of which are usually considerably less than that proposed for Y, have such little influence on the properties of a remedy.

Of course, $[\Gamma\%]_x + [\Gamma\%]_y = 64 + 4 = 68\%$, leaving 32% of molecular memory apparently empty. However, it is not really empty at all, since the 32% contains garbled or unintelligible patterns derived from X and Y. These become overwritten by the coherent geometries of X and Y as potentization progresses from one phase to the next. Thus, a 6c contains less 'garbage information' than a 1c. The LM method of preparation theoretically removes such 'garbage information' more efficiently than the liquid phase centesimal, and the liquid phase centesimal more efficiently than the liquid phase decimal (Lessell, 2002).

Example 2

The point about impurities can be reinforced by considering molecule Y to be such an unwanted impurity, and now adding a third hypothetical molecule Z to the previous bimolecular example, and in the same concentration as X, i.e. 8g/dl. Therefore, $\Sigma A = 18$g/dl. $\Psi_x = 8/18 = 0.44$, so $[\Gamma\%]_x = 100\,(0.44)^2 = 19.36\%$. The same must, of course, apply to $[\Gamma\%]_z$, since Z is present in the same absolute, and thus relative, concentration. And finally we have $\Psi_y = 2/18 = 0.11$, and $[\Gamma\%]_y = 100(0.11)^2 = 1.21\%$. Thus, with regard to the 'desirable' molecules X and Z, their total contribution to imprinting is $[\Gamma\%]_{(x+z)} = [\Gamma\%]_x + [\Gamma\%]_z = 19.36 + 19.36 = 38.72\%$. Hence, $[\Gamma\%]_{(x+z)} / [\Gamma\%]_y = 38.72/1.21 = 32$. Thus, as a result of adding Z, the influence of the impurity Y on molecular memory is now 32 times less than that of its rivals (as compared with 16 times in Example 1). Whilst further stages of potentization will increase the absolute value of $[\Gamma\%]_y$, on a theoretical basis it will always be 32 times less than $[\Gamma\%]_{(x+z)}$, since this too is increased by the same factor.

Of course, any molecule or ion present in minor relative concentration may be classified as either an 'impurity' or a 'minor ingredient'. If it is there by deliberate action, it is a minor ingredient;

if not, it is an impurity. Whatever the case may be, it is poorly represented in molecular memory. Hence, it is really those substances present in significantly larger relative concentrations that call the tune. Indeed, the standardization of mother tinctures should be determined by this fact.

It must also be said that there is some importance to be attached to the strength of a mother tincture destined for potentization. If it does not contain a high total absolute concentration of desirable solutes, then it is more likely to be overwhelmed by the effects of impurities in the diluent. Thus, whilst 1 drop of a good quality mother tincture may be added to 99 drops of diluent to produce the first centesimal potency, a weaker one may require 2 drops to be added to 98, or even 3 to 97. Indeed, the French and German Homeopathic Pharmacopoeiae suggest such precautions as routine (FHP, 1982; GHP, 1990).

In that this mathematical model helps us to explain the fact that minor molecules and ions usually play little part in the making of a remedy, it allows us to understand why tap water with all its impurities can be used, under certain circumstances, for serial dilution (see below, *Fluxion*). The model also allows us to make other predictions of interest, as shown in the examples below.

Example 3

If we were to potentize a simple solution of Na^+Cl^-, would the influence of Na^+ on molecular memory be the same as that of Cl^-? Well, according to our model it would not, since the absolute concentration of each ion must be expressed in terms of weight per unit volume, rather than molar concentration. (The full reason for this is explained in Lessell, 2002.) Since the relative atomic mass of Na^+ is approximately 23 and that of Cl^- is approximately 35.5, and both must be present in equal numbers, it follows that $\Psi_{Na+} = 23/(23 + 35.5) = 0.39$ and $\Psi_{Cl-} = 35.5/(23 + 35.5) = 0.61$. Hence, $[\Gamma\%]_{Na+} = 100(0.39)^2 = 15.21\%$, and $[\Gamma\%]_{Cl-} = 100(0.61)^2 = 37.21\%$. Rather surprisingly, perhaps, the influence of Cl^- is more than twice that of Na^+. This is of some relevance to understanding the biological properties of the remedy *Natrum muriaticum*, since its principal constituent is NaCl.

Example 4

It is useful to compare the theoretical imprinting properties of another salt of the *Natrum* (sodium) group commonly used in homeopathic practice, i.e. Na_2SO_4, known as *Natrum sulphuricum*. On the face of it, you might guess that it has twice as much sodium imprinting capability as *Natrum muriaticum*. However, guesses are one thing, and calculations another. In solution it dissociates into $2Na^+ + SO_4^{2-}$. The relative atomic masses of the component atoms are approximately: Na 23, S 32, O 16. Thus the relative 'ionic mass' of SO_4^{2-} is 96. Therefore, the ratio of Na^+ to SO_4^{2-} by weight is 46:96. By means of calculations along the lines previously given, we arrive at the conclusion that the influence of Na^+ on molecular memory is 10.5% (compared with 15.21% for *Natrum muriaticum*), whilst that of SO_4^{2-} is 45.7%. If nothing else, this indicates that, despite having two rather than one Na^+ ions, a given potency of *Natrum sulphuricum* is less of a conveyer of the sodium 'image' to a biological system than a similarly prepared potency of *Natrum muriaticum*.

Types of energization

Fundamental to the process of imprinting is the delivery of energy, and this can be applied in various ways. These methods may be divided into 'classical' and 'non-classical' on a historical basis, or according to whether they are currently viewed as 'conventional' or 'unconventional', as shown in Figure 2.8.

Classical energization: succussion

Each episode of succussion involves vigorous shaking of a liquid phase preparation, and usually the delivery of a final sharp blow to the vial – classically against a leather-bound book, but a rubber pad may also be used. This blow is applied after each stage of serial dilution. The vial should be of such a size that it is about two-thirds to three-quarters full. For centesimal dilutions, a '5ml' vial (which actually holds about 6ml) can be used to process 4.5ml of diluent.

Succussion may be performed by hand or mechanically (see Figures 2.9 and 2.10), and there is considerable variation between pharmacies in the number of succussions applied per stage of serial dilution, the precise way in which they are carried out, and the total amount of mechanical energy delivered in the process. Defining 'one succussion' as one episode of vigorous agitation plus one forceful blow, the number applied varies from two to 100 for each stage of serial dilution; though two is more of historical significance, and most pharmacists are consistent in their technique or 'house style'. A simple approach to manual succussion without the use of the leather book is as follows (BHP, 1882):

> grasping it [the vial] in the right hand, with the thumb held firmly over the cork, shake it well, letting each shake terminate in a jerk by striking the closed right hand against the open palm of the left hand.

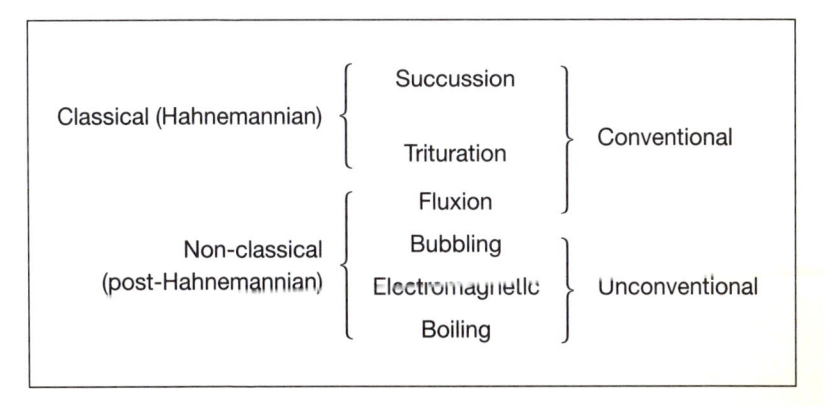

Classical (Hahnemannian)	{ Succussion / Trituration }	Conventional
Non-classical (post-Hahnemannian)	{ Fluxion / Bubbling / Electromagnetic / Boiling }	Unconventional

Figure 2.8
Methods of energization.

Apart from simple mixing of the vial contents, it may be suggested that the object of succussion is to produce 'molecular shearing'. This involves the enforced juxtaposition of electrostatically repulsive ions or the poles of polar molecules, followed by their forcible distraction at right angles to the action of the repulsive force. Rather than just producing heat, it can be proposed that this also leads to the production of an unknown form of energy which is required for the transfer of information concerning molecular and ionic geometry to the diluent, and its progressive intensification. With respect to this energy, it is envisaged that the vial and its

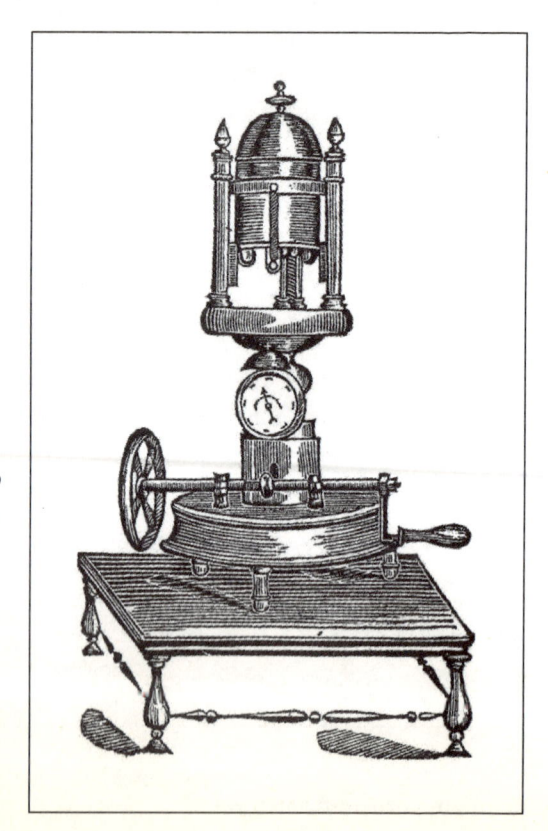

Figure 2.9 Somolinos Mechanical Succussion Apparatus. From the pricelist of La Farmacia Homeopática de Don Cesáreo Martin Somolinos, Madrid, 1866. An early attempt to reduce wear and tear on the pharmacist.

contents act as a type of capacitor. Once a level of 'critical capacitance' has been reached, the stored energy begins to interfere with the imprinting process. As a result, no more informational transfer or intensification can be achieved by further episodes of succussion. This can only be reinstated by discarding a significant amount of the potentized diluent, and then adding fresh alcohol–water. This is why serial dilution is a necessity for progressive imprinting. There is also the possibility that the 'maximal capacitance' is only slightly greater than the 'critical capacitance', so that little more energy is stored in the vial after the latter has been exceeded, with any further episodes of succussion mainly yielding heat.

Whether the 'critical capacitance' is actually reached for each stage of serial dilution depends on four principal factors:

1. The amount of energy remaining in the residue from the previous serial dilution.
2. The total amount of energy delivered.
3. The aggressiveness of delivery.
4. The viscosity of the vial contents.

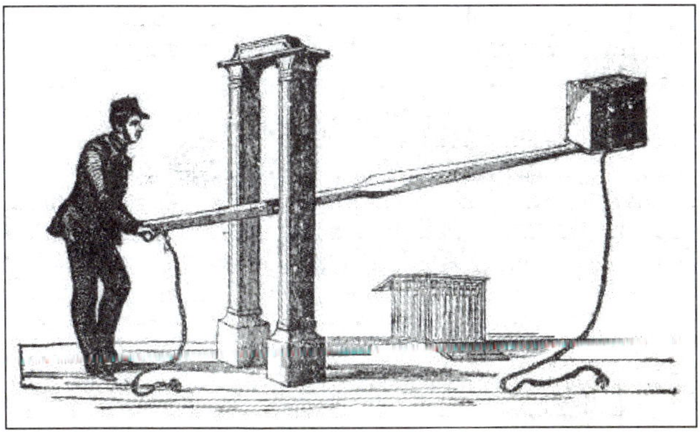

Figure 2.10
Benoît Mure Succussion Machine, *c.* 1838. The first mechanical succussion apparatus. Dr Benoît Mure introduced homeopathy into Brazil and Egypt.

There is some evidence with respect to centesimal dilutions that there is little point in going beyond 60 episodes of hand succussion per dilution (Kayne, 1997). Nevertheless, it is to be noted that LM-scale potencies are routinely prepared using 100 succussions per dilution. That this does not cause the critical capacitance to be exceeded, is quite feasible, since the serial dilution factor of 1 in 50 000 ensures that a much smaller proportion of the contents of the vial and its stored energy is retained after each phase than is the case for remedies prepared on the centesimal scale (serial dilution factor 1 in 100). In other words, assuming that the critical capacitance has been at least closely approached in both cases, the retention of energy from any previous dilution may be in the order of 500 times less for an LM preparation than for a centesimal. In the case of the decimal scale, the rather low dilution factor of 1 in 10 causes critical capacitance to be reached much sooner in comparison with even the centesimal scale. As a result, the decimal scale, as far as *liquid* potencies are concerned, must be regarded as weaker therapeutically than the centesimal (so that D6 is weaker than 6c), although this is probably only of significance with numerical potencies in excess of 30.

If kinetic energy were delivered slowly and gently to a vial over the course of a few minutes, little imprinting or intensification would occur. This is because there would be insufficient molecular shearing to produce the appropriate form of energy. It follows that 'fiercer' potencies result from forceful agitation and sharp blows. Thus, the total amount of energy applied, though relevant, is less important than its mode of delivery – unless, of course, we are in the business of producing weaker remedies. Indeed, 'anthroposphical pharmacy', based on the work of Rudolf Steiner (1861–1925), uses an unusual form of gentle succussion in the production of its serial decimal potencies (see Figure 2.11). Those interested in this subject will note that the philosophy of anthroposophical pharmacy is also somewhat different in other ways, including the selection and treatment of original substances, which are governed by very precise and particular rules.

The viscosity of a liquid phase preparation, though partially affected by any solute, is largely determined by the alcohol content, and to some degree by the temperature. The percentage of ethanol used as a diluent ranges from 20 to 96%. The higher this percentage, the less the viscosity. The less the viscosity, the greater the facilitation of molecular shearing. Hence, alcohol (see Figure 2.12) plays five roles in liquid phase potentization:

1. It acts as a solvent.
2. It facilitates energization.
3. It becomes imprinted with molecular and ionic information.
4. It donates this information to unimprinted diluent molecules.
5. It acts as a preservative.

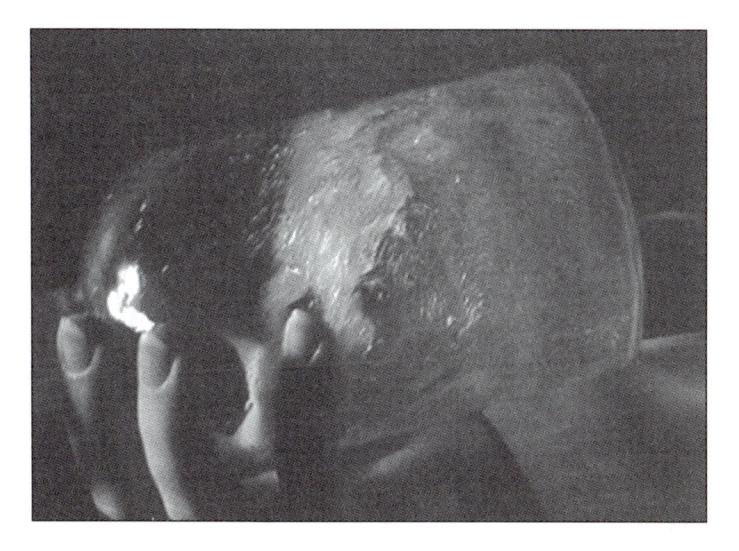

Figure 2.11
Anthroposophical succussion. A large bottle is shaken in a smooth rhythmical manner such as to induce a figure-of-eight pattern, at a rate of about 70 times per minute. Organic substances are succussed for 2.5 minutes, and inorganic for 4. Photograph by courtesy of Weleda (UK) Ltd., Ilkeston.

Classical energization: trituration

Trituration involves the vigorous grinding of an original substance with lactose in a mortar. This is carried out for various lengths of time, in varying ways according to the nature of the original substance, and may be achieved either manually or mechanically (see Figures 2.13–2.18). Serial dilution with lactose is only carried out on either the decimal or centesimal scale, and is based solely on weight (e.g. 1c = 1g in 100g = 1g:99g). In order to facilitate the process, the appropriate amount of lactose for each stage of serial dilution is divided and added in stages (see below).

Trituration is usually reserved for substances insoluble in ethanol–water (e.g. mercury and quartz), but those who wish to adhere strongly to Hahnemann's post-1835 ideas will triturate any

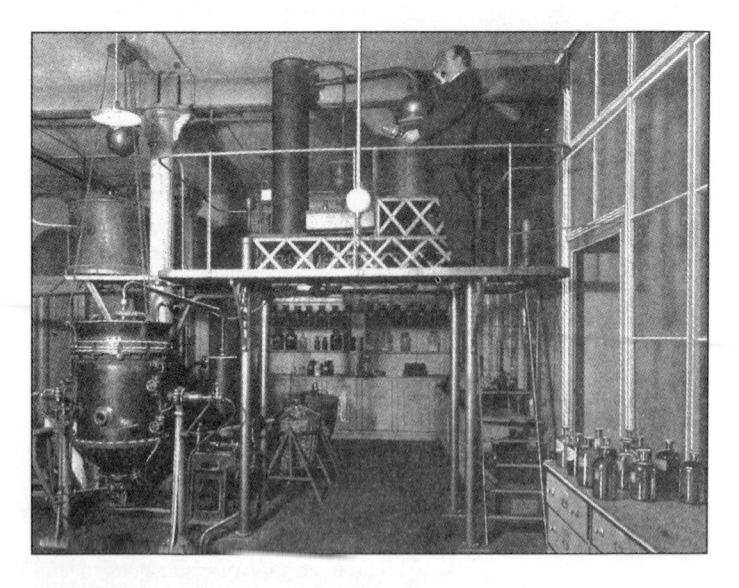

Figure 2.12
Distillation plant for the production of spirits. Homeopathic Central Pharmacy of Dr Willmar Schwabe, Leipzig, *c.* 1920.

material up to a potency of 3c, whether insoluble or not. The fact that the pulverized parts of dried plants may be triturated to produce therapeutically individualized remedies strongly suggests that cellulose itself does not imprint itself on the diluent.

Once a dilution of 1 in 10^6 is achieved, all triturated substances will go into proper solution or colloidal suspension. Thus, there is no need to triturate beyond 3c or D6, and further potentization is carried out in the liquid phase. In this regard, it is worth noting that lactose becomes insoluble where too much alcohol is present. This is why, in Stage 2 of LM manufacture, Hahnemann tells us to use water and 90% alcohol in the ratio of 4:1; and, for Stage 5 onwards, to dissolve a single globule/granule in 1 drop of water before proceeding with the addition of alcohol (see above, *Manufacture of LMs*). As a further example, we may quote his instructions (Hahnemann, 1845) for the processing of a solid phase 3c into a liquid phase 4c (my notes are in square brackets):

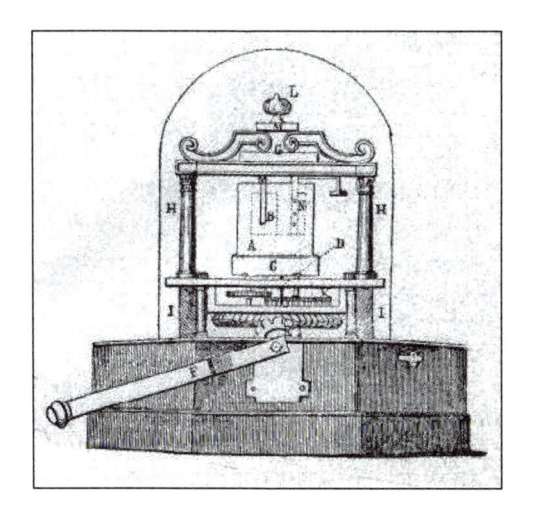

Figure 2.13
Benoît Mure Triturator, *c.* 1838. One of the earliest mechanical devices for producing homogeneous triturations.

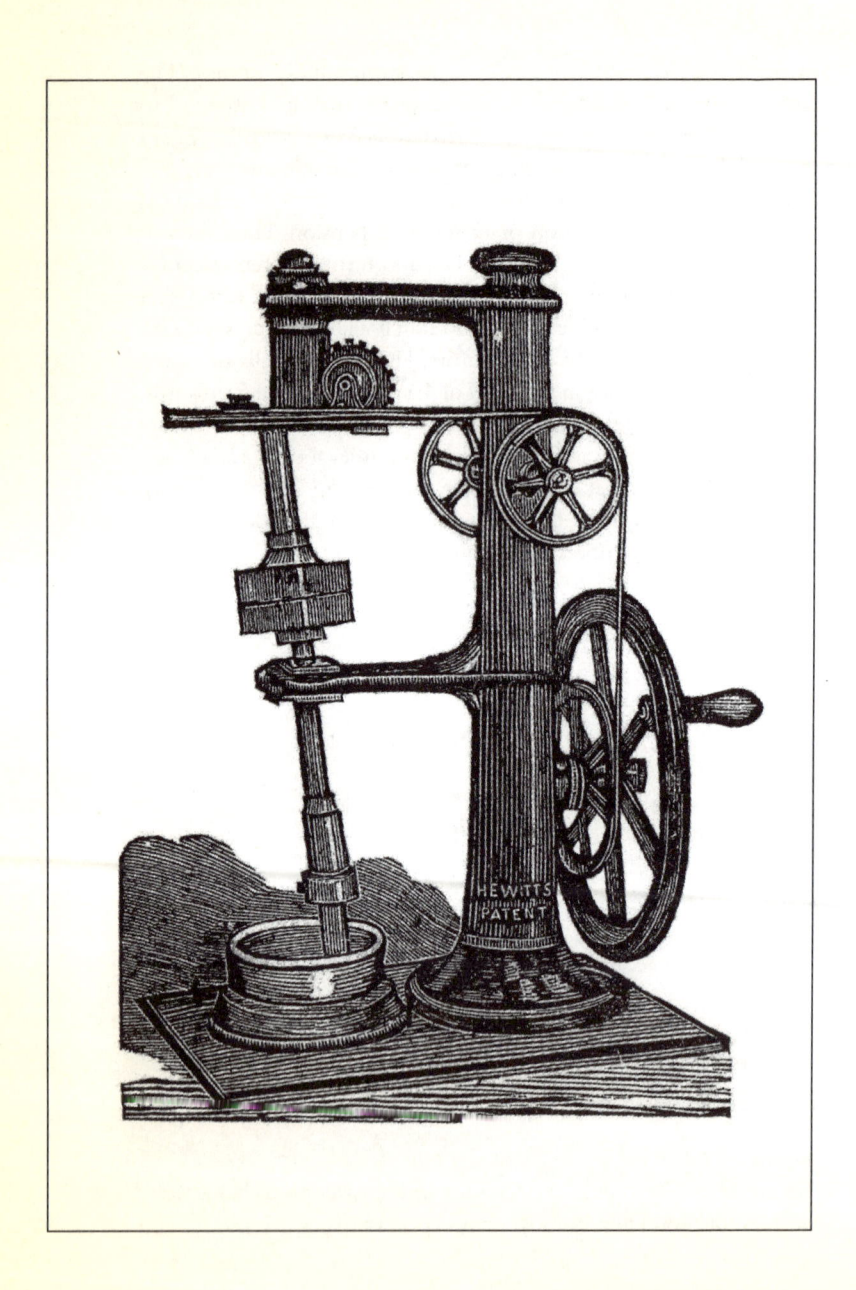

Figure 2.14
Hewitt Mechanical Triturator. From the pricelist of La Farmacia Homeopática de Don Cesáreo Martin Somolinos, Madrid, 1866. The *British Homoeopathic Pharmacopoeia* (2nd edition), 1876, says of this apparatus: 'Several attempts have been made to invent machines for triturating the drugs, some of which are very ingenious, and to a certain extent effective. The best we are acquainted with in this country is that of Mr Hewitt; but even this cannot compete with the human hand: a careful microscopic comparison between machine and hand-made preparations showed conclusively that when the medicinal substance was hard, and in considerable pieces ... Mr Hewitt's machine failed to reduce the particles to the uniformly minute size which was attained in the hand-made triturations; when, however, the medicine was already in pulverulent form ... there appeared little difference between the two modes of triturating.' By the twentieth century, rather more sophisticated devices had been developed, producing results even better than those produced by hand (see Figures 2.15–2.18). Hahnemann Laboratories of the USA currently use a 'ball mill', consisting of a cylindrical porcelain jar with a tight lid containing small carborundum cylinders (the 'balls'). The jar is rotated continuously by means of a pair of horizontal motorized rollers.

> To one [Nuremberg] grain [62mg] of the millionth trituration [3c] you add 50 drops of distilled water, and turn the vial several times around its axis. By this means the sugar of milk becomes dissolved. Then you add 50 drops of good alcohol [95%], and shake the vial [dilution: 1 grain in 100 drops or about 4.5ml].

These days, however, the pharmacist is more likely to secure a 1g in 100ml dilution by adding 0.04g (40mg) of the 3c trituration to 4ml of a diluent of low alcohol content. However, in some pharmacies, where the 4c is to be medicated on solid forms, for which a high alcohol content is required, the diluent used is 95% alcohol (see Chapter 4, *Liquid potencies*). Under such circumstances, lactose itself is almost insoluble – but it would appear that the medicinal imprint is still sufficiently transferred to the highly alcoholic diluent for it to become therapeutically active, and

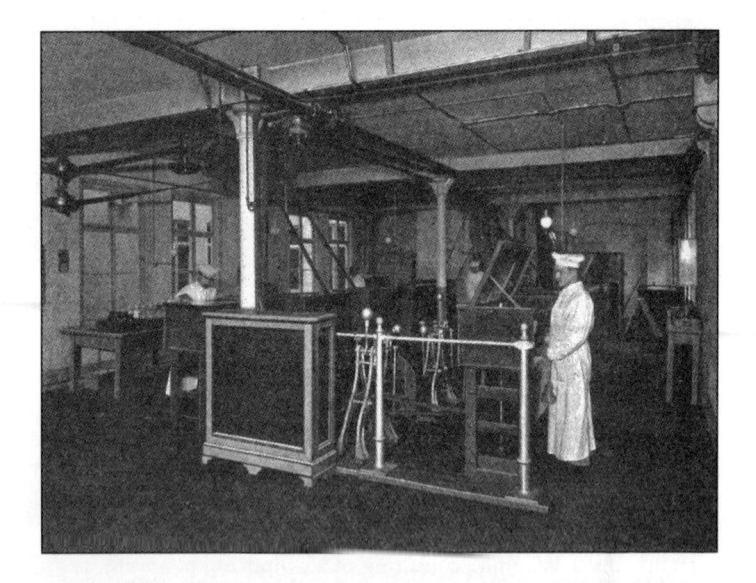

Figure 2.15
Trituration Machine. Homeopathic Central Pharmacy of Dr Willmar Schwabe, Leipzig, *c.* 1920.

After 10 minutes.

After 20 minutes.

After 30 minutes.

After 40 minutes.

After 50 minutes.

After 60 minutes.

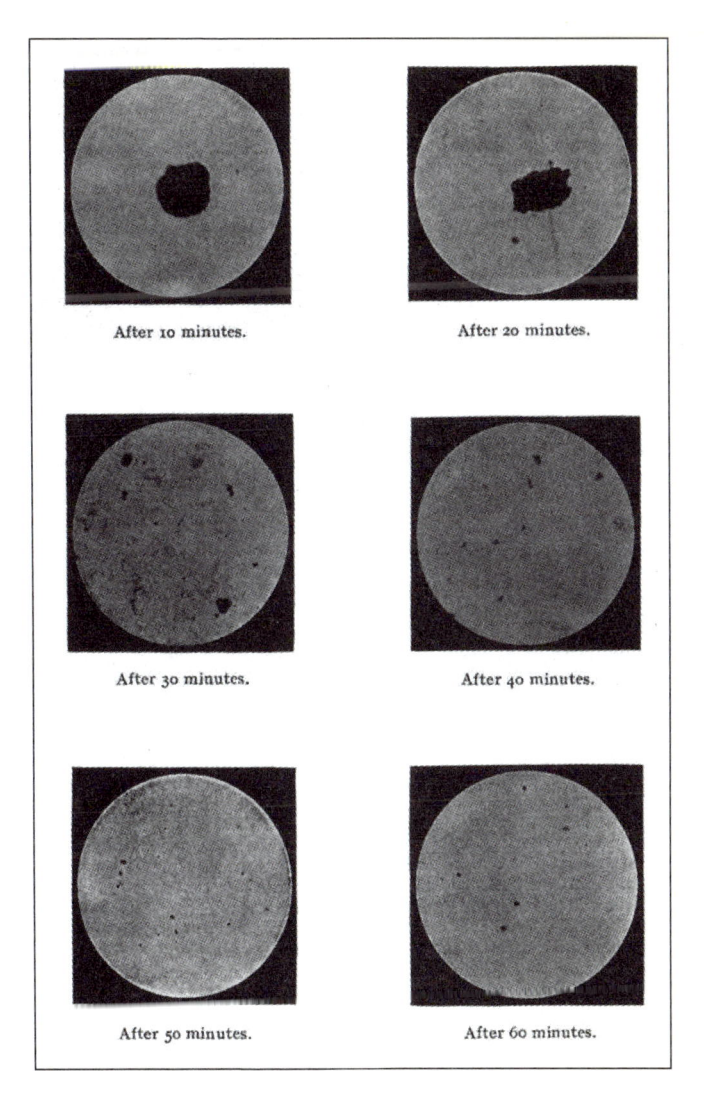

Figure 2.16
Microscopy of handmade trituration of *Cuprum metallicum* (copper) D1. Magnification: 180×.

Figure 2.17
Microscopy of *Cuprum metallicum* (copper) D1 after 60 minutes of trituration with the Dr Willmar Schwabe machine (see Figure 2.15).

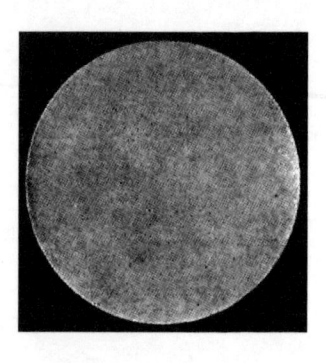

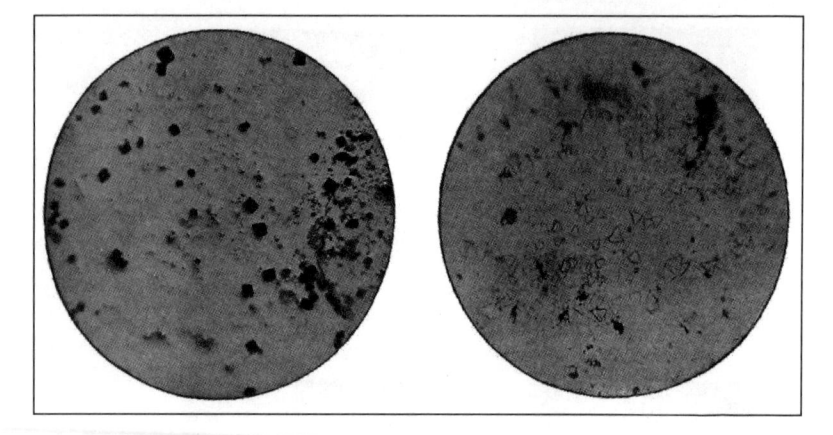

Figure 2.18
Microscopy of trituration. *Left*: Evidence of copper from *Cuprum aceticum* (copper acetate) D5 (1 in 100 000). Magnification: 220×. *Right*: Evidence of salt from *Natrum muriaticum* (rock salt) D7 (1 in 10 000 000). Magnification: 220×.

this may even be used subsequently to produce a 5c potency of satisfactory quality. The transfer of information results from the leaching of imprinted water and lactose molecules from the triturated material.

To continue on this theme, we should now examine how a solid phase D6 is converted into a liquid phase D7. In the nineteenth century (BHP, 1882), this was achieved by first adding 10 Troy grains (10 × 65mg = 650mg) of the triturated material to 95 minims ('standard drops') of water plus 5 of 95% alcohol (100 minims in total). This was left for a few hours, occasionally agitated, and then followed by proper succussion. The dilution was thus 1 grain in 10 minims. However, a more modern 1g in 10ml dilution may be achieved by dissolving 0.4g (400mg) of the D6 trituration in 4ml of weak alcohol.

The principles involved in imprinting are similar to those for liquid phase potentization, including the matter of critical capacitance. However, the level of contamination with atmospheric and vessel wall impurities is probably higher – not that this makes much difference to a properly prepared remedy (see above, *Impurities*). More importantly, the process of trituration is mechanically inefficient, and a large amount of energy must be applied to break up the original substance and grains of lactose, this being mainly dissipated as heat. In fact, the ability of the process to produce satisfactory imprinting depends less on the limitations of critical capacitance than it does on its capacity for the mechanical disruption of solids.

An extract from the third edition of the *British Homoeopathic Pharmacopoeia* (BHP, 1882) considers the process of trituration in some considerable detail. In comparing centesimal scale trituration with decimal, it indicates that the latter method is more mechanically advantageous (my additions are in square brackets):

> This form of preparation was originally designed by Hahnemann, who published minute directions as to how it should be performed. His method is still adhered to, and there is only one alteration which may with advantage be made, and that is in the proportion of sugar of milk [lactose] to be used at each stage of the process. Hahnemann recommends 1 [Nuremberg] grain [62mg] of the substance to be triturated with 99 grains of sugar of milk, and the process lasts one hour. It is, however, preferable to use the proportion of 1 [Troy] grain

[65mg] of medicine to 9 of sugar of milk, and in this way each decimal trituration after the first [which takes 60 minutes] will occupy forty minutes, or each centesimal – being equal to two decimal triturations – to the making of which Hahnemann allotted one hour, will now occupy [at least] one hour and twenty minutes. The object of this change is chiefly to insure [sic] a more thorough preparation, it being found by the microscope that the addition of so large a proportion of sugar of milk at one time (33 grains to 1 grain of medicine) renders it more difficult to reduce the size of the particles of medicine, especially if they are hard, and thus deteriorates the value of trituration. Since Hahnemann avowedly invented this process for the purpose of reducing the drug to the finest possible powder, the modification proposed is merely carrying out his own ideas to a higher degree of perfection.

For the first decimal trituration the steps of the process are as follows: Weigh any number of grains (not exceeding 100 grains) of the medicinal substance, which should be in a fine powder, or, in the case of some metals, in thin leaf, and then weigh separately an equal number of grains of perfectly pure sugar of milk in coarse powder. Transfer the medicinal substance into a perfectly clean and dry Wedgwood mortar, and then place the milk sugar upon it. And mix the two together with a horn or ivory spatula [Hahnemann recommends porcelain], or, in the case of metallic leaf [e.g. gold], spread the milk sugar evenly over the surface. Using a pestle of the same material as the mortar, rub the mixture thoroughly and carefully during six minutes, taking care that it should only be mixed thoroughly by the steady circular movement so well known to pharmaceutists in mixing powders, but also that the hard, grinding motion which is employed in incorporating pill-mass [almost a lost art] should be effectively used, so as to break up all large and hard particles. At the end of the six minutes, scrape the pestle and mortar carefully with the spatula, so that nothing shall be left adhering to them and stir the mixture again – a process which will occupy about four minutes. Again rub and stir the mixture with the pestle for six minutes as before, and again scrape all the particles off the mortar and pestle, and thus complete the first stage of the process.

As the reducing of the medicine to the finest possible powder is a most essential point in the method of preparation, and as it is very difficult to effect this after a large proportion of sugar of milk has been added, a small portion of the trituration should be carefully examined under the microscope at this stage, and if the particles are found to be unequal in size, the trituration and scraping should be continued until the reduction of the particles to a uniform degree of fineness is complete. Now add three times as many grains of coarsely-powdered sugar of milk★ as were used in the first instance, and stir it well in with the triturated material, and proceed as before, – viz., rubbing for six minutes, scraping and mixing for four minutes, again rubbing for six minutes, and scraping as above. Then add five times the number of grains used first, of finely-powdered sugar of milk, rub for six minutes, scrape and mix for four minutes, and again rub for six minutes, after which the trituration may be viewed as complete, and having once more scraped the whole together, it should be transferred to a perfectly clean, dry, glass bottle, and labelled as 1^x [1x, D1].

For subsequent triturations the steps are as follows: Take one part by weight (not exceeding 100 grains) of the previous trituration, and then weigh separately nine times as many grains of perfectly pure sugar of milk in fine powder. Transfer half of the quantity of the sugar of milk into a mortar as above, then place the triturated substance on the sugar of milk, and mix the two together with a horn or ivory spatula. Rub the mixture as directed for six minutes, scrape the mortar and pestle carefully with a spatula, so that nothing is left adhering to them. Again rub the mixture with the pestle for six minutes as before, and again scrape and mix thoroughly, when the first stage of the process is complete. Now add the remainder of the sugar of

---

★In the case of metallic leaf it may be necessary to add a little of this second quantity of coarse milk sugar before all the particles can be brought under the pestle; in this case the smallest quantity should be added at a time, so as to avoid increasing the bulk materially, before perfect reduction of the metal is secured.

milk, stir it well with the triturated material, and proceed as before – viz., rubbing for six minutes, scraping and mixing for four minutes, and again rubbing for six minutes, after which the pestle and mortar may be scraped, and the triturated product bottled, corked, and labelled.

In consequence of the extreme difficulty with which pestles and mortars can be cleaned to the degree necessary for our refined processes, all careful homoeopathic chemists procure perfectly new ones for each substance and then label them in the name of the medicine, and never use them for any other purpose; and even, notwithstanding this, it is necessary to be very careful in the thorough washing and cleaning of the apparatus [Hahnemann himself recommended: wash in hot water, dry, then boil in water for 30 minutes, or set on glowing coals].

It should be noted that triturated material is not always 'upgraded' to a higher liquid potency, and may, indeed, be dispensed as such (see Chapter 4, *Triturated material*).

Fluxion

Fluxion is actually both a method of energization and one of serial dilution. Its use is essentially restricted to mechanical devices for the production of very high potencies from liquid phase preparations of not less than 12c. In the Pinkus Potentizer (developed at Ainsworths Pharmacy, London), a jet of deionized water is injected into a stainless steel vial under some pressure. Using the Korsakovian principle, only one such vial is required, and this is emptied each time by means of suction. This particular machine also delivers successive blows to the vial at each stage of serial dilution.

The important thing to point out is that large quantities of air bubbles can be injected with some force during the process of automatic fluxion. Indeed, according to the water pressure, this may be sufficient to cause them to enter that important marginal zone adjacent to the inner wall of the vial. Under the circumstances, it might be thought that the atmospheric gases would be potentized themselves. However, to do this, they must compete with the existing molecular memories inherited from the starting liquid potency (12c in the Pinkus method). It would appear that, by the time a potency of 5–12c has been reached, molecular memory is sufficiently occupied with information concerning the original substance to block the acquisition of much else (though such information concerning the original substance can be intensified further). Furthermore, it is likely that this state of affairs is transferred to any new molecules of diluent entering the system, thus preventing them also from taking the imprint of those gases to any significant degree.

On a historical note, it should be mentioned that a fluxion device was patented as early as 1869 by Bernard Fincke. A later device, using fluxion with tap water, and developed by Thomas Skinner (1825–1906), is perhaps better known (see Figure 2.19), a modified form of which is still in current use.

Bubbling and prepotentization

It might be thought that the transfer of medicinal geometry to a liquid diluent starts with succussion of the first serial dilution. However, we might imagine that a mother tincture which has been shaken repeatedly in the course of its manufacture may be subject to a similar transfer of solute geometry to the solvent. Thus, when it is dispersed in ethanol–water to create the first dilution, even before being properly energized, the formation of an appropriate imprint on the diluent has already been initiated, albeit to a minor degree. In this way, herbal remedies given in liquid form may have slightly different clinical properties from those given as a tablet.

This phenomenon, which we may term 'prepotentization', is also of relevance to the preparation of homoeopathic remedies from relatively insoluble gases, such as argon, where their presence in solution may be overshadowed by that of other gases and various impurities. However, in order to prepare such a gas for classical potentization, it must first of all be bubbled through the diluent for a few minutes. Since this, in itself, is a form of mechanical energization of the minute bubbles which pass through the diluent,

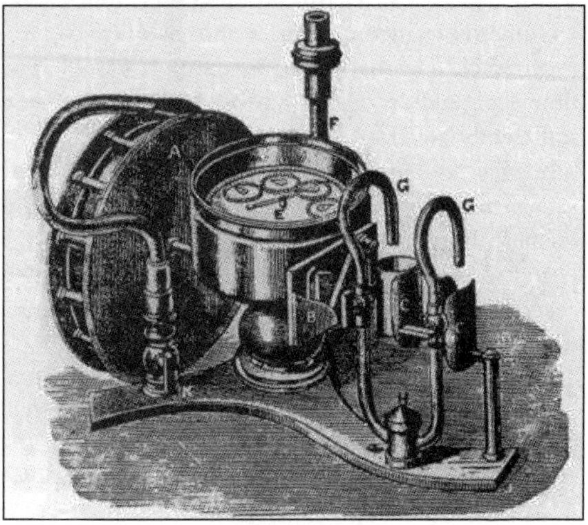

Figure 2.19
The Skinner Fluxion Centesimal Potentizer/Attenuator, *c.* 1878. This apparatus used mains tap water both as a source of power and as a diluent.

Key
A: Water wheel of 15cm diameter, providing the motive power, and regulated by a stopcock **K**.
B: Mechanical rack and slot mechanism for alternately tipping and restoring the vial cradles **C, C**.
E: Series of dials to register the number of episodes of serial potentization.
F: Water inlet pipe attached to house/pharmacy main.
G, G: Phosphor-bronze jets to discharge water into the glass vials. Attached via an isolating stopcock to the coupling **H**, usually only one jet **G** was in use, together with one glass vial (as illustrated). Although the discharge of water via **G** was continuous in automatic mode, the apparatus was adjusted so that the vial was regularly tipped out when the water level reached its brim. However, the machine was not put fully into this mode until a 5th centesimal potency had been achieved by partially manual operation. Moreover, hand successions were applied to the 1c, 4c and 5c potencies. Where any particular potency was to be stored for clinical use (e.g. 30c, 200c), the final stage of potentization was carried out manually, using alcohol-water (as is still the case with modern aqueous fluxion techniques). The machine was capable of producing 50 centesimal potencies per minute, 3000 per hour, 72 000 per day, 100 000 in about 33 hours, and one million in about 14.5 days, running day and night.

and is also of sufficient strength to cause them to enter that important marginal zone in significant quantities, we can assume that the imprint of the geometry of the gas on the diluent begins at this stage. Furthermore, there is a distinct possibility that the surplus gas leaving the system carries with it excesses of energy accumulating in the diluent, so that critical capacitance is not achieved, with its adverse effect on imprinting. In exhibiting this property, bubbling is rather like serial dilution, and imprinting and intensification of molecular and ionic imagery may continue for the entire duration of the process. Thus, when we arrive at the first serial dilution, the process of imprinting is expanded mainly from diluent molecules carrying the memory of that gas, rather than from the small quantity of gas that is actually in solution.

This, of course, is quite different from the situation that prevails with fluxion, where the gases must compete with an inherited imprint of relatively high intensity (see above, *Fluxion*).

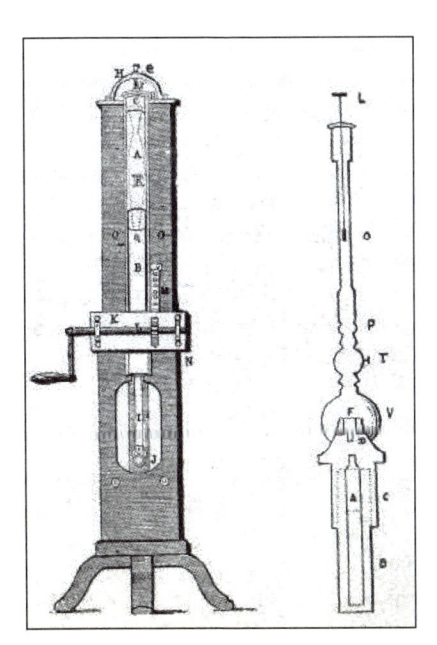

Figure 2.20
Benoît Mure Vacuum Device, c. 1838. This apparatus 'to create a vacuum' was presumably to eliminate air from the potentizing vial. No-one since seems to have pursued the matter.

Electromagnetic energization

It is fairly well known that sunlight will gradually destroy potentized homeopathic remedies. It is perhaps strange to learn, therefore, that sunlight can also be used to produce remedies. Indeed, we might say 'he who giveth also taketh away'. Both phenomena are attributable to the ultraviolet wavelengths of sunlight.

The sun energization method is of spagyric origin. In homeopathic pharmacy, its use is confined to the preparation of Bach and other Flower Remedies. In the Bach method, living blooms are floated on water and exposed to solar radiation for 3 hours. During this process, which extracts some chemical substances from the flowers, their characteristic vital electromagnetic field pattern is also transferred to water molecules, whilst the achievement of critical capacitance is probably avoided by energy loss via evaporation. The flowers are then removed. The remaining liquid is vigorously shaken with an equal quantity of grape brandy (dilution: 1 in 2). It is then further diluted to 1 in 10^5 with 22% ethanol and some agitation. Because they are prepared in an unconventional manner, there is some dispute as to whether the Flower Remedies are truly homeopathic or not. However, in that they rely on the imprinting of diluent molecules for their effect, they must be deemed to be so. Indeed, imprinting and intensification are actually associated with one stage of sun energization and two of the mechanical kind. Nevertheless, claims that the 1 in 10^5 dilution is essentially the same as a D5 (5x) prepared more conventionally are difficult to support. If anything, they would appear to be stronger, this being due to the efficiency of sun energization itself.

Sunlight only depotentizes remedies where the original substance is either completely or very nearly absent. As we have seen with the Flower Remedies, provided the original material is present in significant quantities, it is a useful means of energization.

When vials of ethanol–water are exposed to a variety of electromagnetic phenomena for varying lengths of time, the diluent becomes imprinted with their characteristics. This is yet another example of prepotentization (see above, *Bubbling and prepotentization*), and such vials can then be subjected to normal serial dilution and

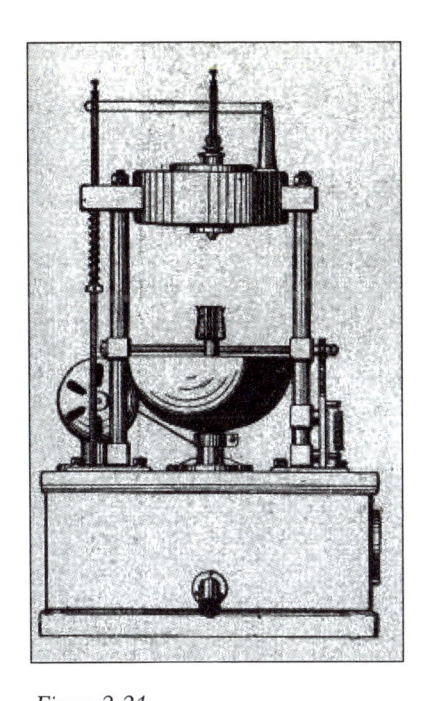

Figure 2.21
Perdrisat-Nebel Automatic Potentizer, early twentieth century.
The desire to accelerate the production of homeopathic remedies rapidly led homeopaths to develop mechanical equipment. As early as 1838, Benoît Mure (1809–1858) built a triturator (Figure 2.13), a succussion machine (Figure 2.10), and a device 'to create a vacuum' (Figure 2.20). Later in the nineteenth century, Hewitt (Figure 2.14), Weber (Figure 2.22), Somolinos (Figure 2.9) and Skinner (Figure 2.19) developed devices of various types. In Switzerland, the engineer Perdrisat of Geneva, in consultation with Antoine Nebel (1870–1954), created an automatic liquid phase potentizer utilizing serial Korsakovian dilutions (see illustration above). In Germany, Schwabe participated in the production of numerous apparatuses (Figure 2.15). In France, the pharmacist René Baudry (1880–1966) also contributed to the development of several devices, principally in collaboration with Perdrisat, but also with Léon Vannier (1880–1963).

succussion. The imprinted phenomena include such things as magnetic fields, sunlight, x-rays and VDU emissions. These are probably recorded by the clouds of virtual photons that enshroud the electrons of the diluent molecules. These photons continually arise from the zero point field (see Chapter 3, *Van der Waals' forces and the Casimir effect*). The actual imprinting process may involve a substitution of real photons for virtual ones, or the impression of a new magnetic field pattern on their own. Since, however, this photonic field is used to energize the electron, thereby preventing its collapse into the nucleus, any such imprints disappear with the course of time. Only by subjecting the diluent to routine potentization can an electromagnetic imprint be preserved and intensified.

Electromagnetic energization via magnetic fields is also used in the production of potentized remedies by means of various unconventional apparatuses, such as the Rae card potentizer. The results are said to be comparable to those of more conventionally prepared remedies, but there are, nevertheless, some subtle differences.

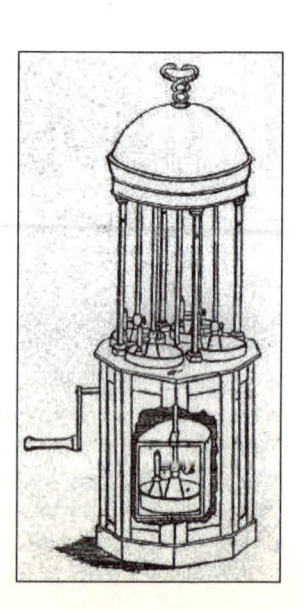

Figure 2.22
Weber Potentizer, nineteenth century.

Boiling

Some of the Bach Flower Remedies are prepared by boiling the plant material in water for 30 minutes. Initial energization occurs only in the subsequent cooling stage from energy stored in the diluent, since boiling itself destroys potentized remedies (see below, *Erasure of imprinting*). As with sun energization, the achievement of critical capacitance is probably avoided by energy loss via evaporation. Again, the resultant liquid is diluted with grape brandy and 22% ethanol as described above. Since boiling kills the plant material, its vital electromagnetic pattern is not imprinted. However, as it is such a potent means of extracting the chemical components, these are imprinted and intensified to a significant degree against any impurities which may be present within the plant material itself or the diluent.

Erasure of imprinting

Potentized remedies are extremely stable and may last for many years. There are, however, a number of things which will 'depotentize' them and thus reduce or eliminate their clinical efficacy. These are:

1. ultraviolet light
2. intense magnetic fields
3. intense x-radiation
4. intense dry heat (120°C or above)
5. intense wet heat (70°C or above).

It has already been remarked that ultraviolet light can have an adverse effect on potentized remedies (see above, *Electromagnetic energization*). Despite the fact that ordinary glass tends to absorb UV radiation, it would seem that the wall of a glass vial is of insufficient thickness to offer complete protection. However, and perhaps perversely, where significant quantities of original substance remain in a low potency liquid phase preparation that has not been medicated on a solid form (see Chapter 4, *Liquid potencies*), there is the theoretical possibility that the penetration of UV light will produce further imprinting and intensification of the molecular memory of the diluent (although, if evaporation is prevented by a tight stopper, then the achievement of critical capacitance will limit the degree to which this occurs; see above, *Electromagnetic energization*).

Though a weak or moderate background magnetic field appears to be essential for potentization to occur, and remedies can even be made from magnetic fields, the presence of intense magnetism not only destroys the potency of remedies (Benveniste, 1994), it also prevents proper imprinting of the diluent. Hence, remedies should be neither prepared nor stored in areas subject to enhanced magnetic effects, such as those associated with electric motors.

Low-intensity x-rays generally present no particular problem, and remedies can even be made from them. Properly controlled airport x-rays are usually of insufficient strength to inactivate remedies, though where there is some doubt, remedies may be placed in x-ray-proof film canisters, available from most photographic stores.

The action of intense dry or wet heat, whilst unimportant under normal circumstances, is advantageous to the pharmacist who wishes to cleanse his equipment of any imprinted residue. Thus mortars, pestles, spatulas and vials may be subjected to either of these techniques after thorough normal cleansing, first with tap water, then with distilled water. Boiling (preferably in distilled water) for 30 minutes, or dry heat at 150°C for 8 hours, should suffice. However, 120°C for about 10 minutes appears to be adequate for any stainless steel vessels.

Another 'enemy of potentization', but in a different way from the others, is the use of plant material mother tinctures that are past their sell-by date. Their chemical composition may have sufficiently altered to affect the properties of any potentized remedy made from them. Most tinctures should be discarded 2 years after manufacture.

Preparatory vessels

Vials may be made of soda or neutral (borosilicate) glass. Soda glass produces a better stable marginal zone (see above, *Impurities*) by virtue of its negative charge, which attracts cations and polar molecules (Lessell, 1994), thus making it better for active potentization. On the other hand, neutral glass is better for long-term storage. Plastic is only permissible for 'emergency potentization', and there is some doubt as to whether it is suitable for the storage of liquid potencies for longer than a few months. Vials in modern fluxion devices may be made of stainless steel. Mortars may be made of any ceramic material or any metal other than iron or plain steel, since these are readily subject to corrosion and the excessive supply of such impurity to the triturated material. The same applies to pestles and spatulas.

Medication of solid forms

Although liquid potencies may be dispensed as such, they are more frequently medicated on various solid forms. This is discussed in Chapter 4, together with posology (dosage) and some further aspects of storage.

The often quoted 'clathrate hydrate theory' suggests that the shape of a molecule or ion of solute is impressed on the diluent through its encagement by hydrogen-bonded clustered molecules of water, these clusters persisting long after the captive molecule or ion has disappeared through progressive dilution. However, whilst there is experimental evidence that 'splashing water' can produce such clathrates (Anagnostatos et al., 1998), they can only be of possible relevance to liquid phase preparations, as they are completely absent in the production of remedies by dry trituration! On this basis alone, the proponents of this theory have surely cut their own throats with Occam's Razor, and it would be wise for us to reject their ideas.

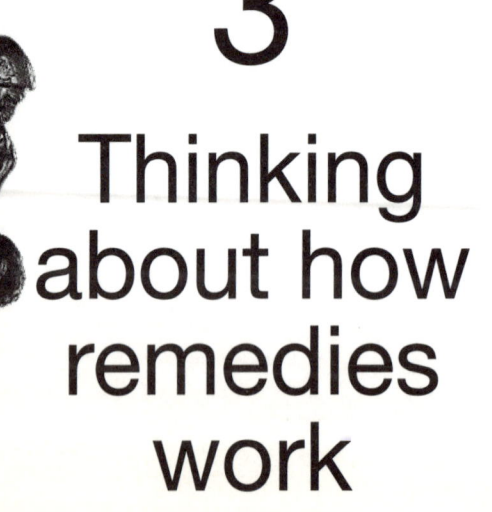

3
Thinking about how remedies work

Introduction

The terms **pharmacodynamics** – the action of drugs on a living system – and **pharmacokinetics** – the action of a living system on drugs – are equally applicable to homeopathic remedies in their potentized form. Nevertheless, whilst the pharmacodynamics of potentized remedies may be viewed as having some close similarities with that of drugs in general, the pharmacokinetics must, because of the remedies' more nebulous nature (see Figure 3.1), be somewhat different.

The process of **potentization**, which involves a number of episodes of serial dilution plus the delivery of mechanical energy after each such episode (see Figure 3.2), is peculiar to homeopathic pharmaceutics. There are, as we have seen in Chapter 2, three scales of serial dilution: the decimal (1 in 10), the centesimal (1 in 100) and the LM or Q (1 in 50 000). Solid phase potentization is achieved by trituration with lactose, whilst liquid phase potentization utilizes alcohol–water (or, less commonly, water alone) as the diluent, and succussion or fluxion (jetting) as the means of energization. This is believed to result in the transfer of information concerning the molecular or ionic imagery of the original substance (e.g. mother tincture solute) to the diluent (alcohol, water, lactose), where it is recorded electromagnetically in an encoded form, perhaps both digitally and holographically – hence, the term 'molecular memory'. In this respect, it is thought that the negative representations of the external geometries of the various molecules and ions of that original substance are transferred individually to the diluent, though with certain exceptions (see Chapter 2, *Diluents*), and to varying degrees according to their relative concentration (see Chapter 2, *Impurities*). In this way, the resultant remedy becomes a conglomerate of such negative geometrical information. It is further proposed that, on administration, this information is pharmacokinetically 'extracted' and amplified, particularly by sites in relation to the mouth, pharynx, and nasal passages, after which it appears as a holographic interference pattern in the magnetic field component of the general electromagnetic field of the body. Since the cells of the body can produce coherent photons (biophotons), it is quite feasible for this hologram to be subject to their projective properties, with the consequent development of real three-dimensional images – these being true representations of the surface geometries of the original molecules or ions from which the remedy was derived, though usually in a negative manner.

In consequence, a homeopathic remedy, as manifest *in vivo*, may present as a magnetic hologram, its photonic projection, or both. The projection is a more architectural field, the conformation of which comprises the overt negative surface geometries of the individual molecules or ions from which it has been derived, just as the faces of the minter's dies depict coins. It may be further suggested that, under certain particular circumstances, some or all of these negative forms are occasionally inverted to positives indirectly, via a pharmacokinetic effect on the magnetic hologram itself. That is to say, each becomes like the coin, rather than the die from which it is struck. It is maintained that it is only the surface configuration of molecules or ions, as determined by their electronic orbitals, and how that is portrayed by the derivative remedy – either negatively or positively, either as a hologram or its projection – that must be regarded as relevant to any homeopathic effect. Polar or ionic charges are thought not to be represented. So, from the pharmacodynamic standpoint, remedies as manifest in the living system are to be regarded as uncharged, despite the fact that they may be transferred to that system via polar molecules, such as water.

In accordance with these propositions, and on a holographically projective basis, a simple geometrical theory is outlined in Part One of this chapter. The theory explains how potentized homeopathic remedies may function at biological receptor sites (Type I action), and some additional proposals concerning their subsequent pharmacokinetic fate are made. For the sake of clarity, this theory is prefaced by a general discussion of drug–receptor interactions, including some new interpretations. Also incorporated in Part One is an explanation of the mechanism by which material doses of a drug may act when selected for any case in the homeopathic manner, i.e. on the basis of the 'Similia Principle' or 'Law of Similars', rather than on allopathic (conventional) grounds. To recapitulate, this principle essentially states that, if a drug D produces

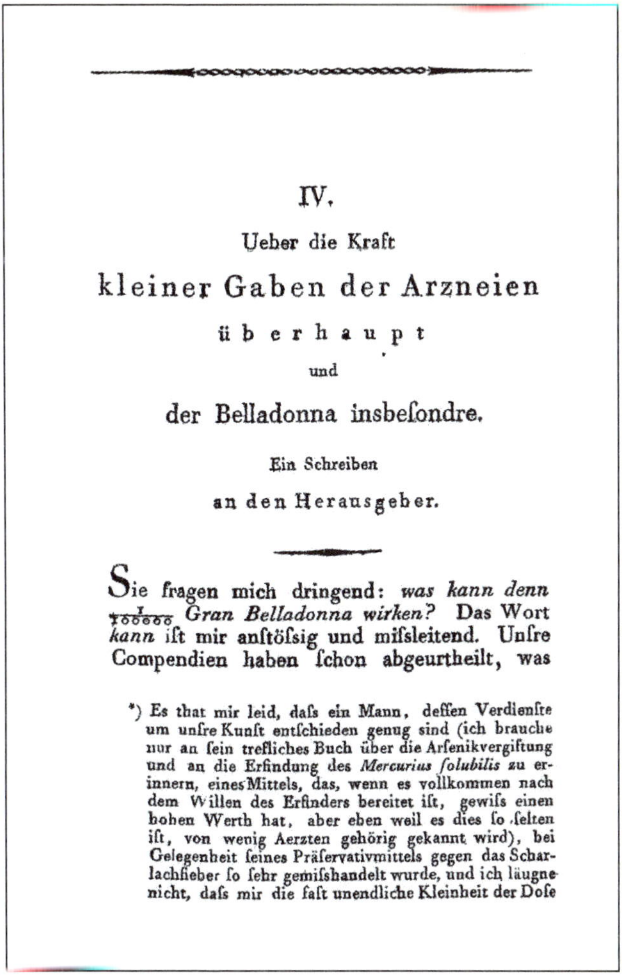

IV.

Ueber die Kraft

kleiner Gaben der Arzneien

überhaupt

und

der Belladonna insbesondre.

Ein Schreiben

an den Herausgeber.

Sie fragen mich dringend: *was kann denn* $\frac{1}{1000000}$ *Gran Belladonna wirken?* Das Wort *kann* ist mir anstöfsig und mifsleitend. Unfre Compendien haben fchon abgeurtheilt, was

*) Es that mir leid, dafs ein Mann, deffen Verdienfte um unfre Kunft entfchieden genug sind (ich brauche nur an fein trefliches Buch über die Arfenikvergiftung und an die Erfindung des *Mercurius folubilis* zu erinnern, eines Mittels, das, wenn es vollkommen nach dem Willen des Erfinders bereitet ift, gewifs einen hohen Werth hat, aber eben weil es dies fo felten ift, von wenig Aerzten gehörig gekannt wird), bei Gelegenheit feines Präfervativmittels gegen das Scharlachfieber fo fehr gemifshandelt wurde, und ich läugne nicht, dafs mir die faft unendliche Kleinheit der Dofe

Figure 3.1
'On the power of small doses of medicine in general, and of Belladonna in particular.' Title page of Hahnemann's early description of the use of *Belladonna* and other drugs in infinitesimal doses, 1801 (Berlin, Hufeland's journal).

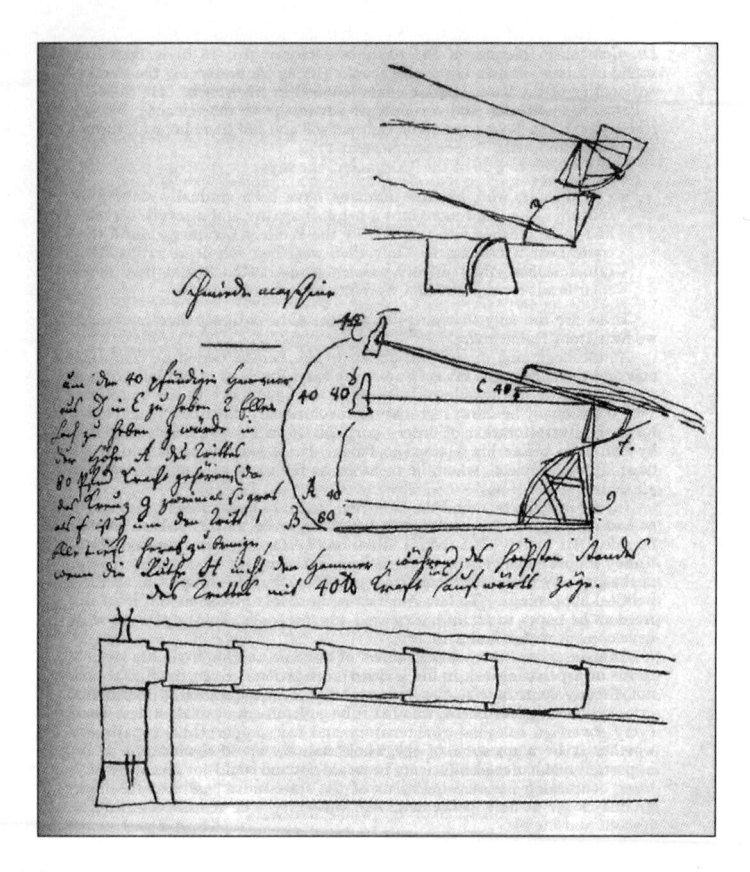

Figure 3.2
Pen sketches by Hahnemann, displaying an interest in successive blows.

physiological effects resembling a certain disease X in a healthy subject, then D may be used to treat a sick person suffering from X. Whilst the homeopathic application of material doses of drugs might seem to be more of historical interest, as it has long since been largely abandoned, it does in fact lend significant support for the notion that homeopathic effects in general, be they produced by material or potentized remedies, are at least partially due to receptor-mediated actions.

In Part Two of this chapter, and as an extension to this theory, it is postulated that a potentized remedy may exert another type of effect on the physiology. Though not involving projection of its hologram or interaction with conventional receptors, the proposed mechanism (Type II action) may be viewed in a geometrical way closely allied to that described for those sites.

It is further suggested that infinitesimal homeopathic remedies may display either or both of these types of action (I and/or II) in any given clinical situation. One important justification for these two models lies in their conjoint ability to explain and connect the various clinical and experimental observations which have accumulated over the last 200 years or so.

Part One
Receptor-mediated action of remedies (Type I action)

Pharmacodynamic docking and locking

In conventional pharmacology, as opposed to classical chemistry, a **ligand** is taken to be any chemical substance D (or part of D) which binds to a biological macromolecular receptor R. D may be a drug, a hormone, a neurotransmitter, a growth factor, an autacoid (e.g. histamine, an angiotensin, a prostaglandin) or an exogenous toxin (e.g. a poison, a bacterial endotoxin or exotoxin). In a sense, all poisons are drugs.

Most receptors are proteins or polypeptides, including enzymes, but some are nucleic acids. Many **drug receptors** are to be found in cellular membranes, where their normal function is to bind endogenous regulatory ligands, such as hormones and neurotransmitters. It is believed that, in general, the primary cause of the association between D and R is geometrical, i.e. that some greater or lesser part of D must fit into some part of R with reasonable accuracy (Katzung, 2001). For convenience, we shall call these parts pD and pR respectively. From the mechanical perspective, this is a lock and key or male and female relationship. This may be termed **coarse geometrical interaction** or **docking**. Furthermore, any given molecule D may have several different zones of pD, each one matching a specific variety of pR.

The attraction of pD to pR is often achieved by ionic or polar attraction. However, the final positional stabilization or 'locking' may involve a number of different chemical interactions. Apart from ionic and hydrogen bonding, which are also associated with attraction, there are van der Waals' forces, hydrophobic interactions and, in relatively rare instances, even covalent bonds. With the exception of covalent bonding (as typified by the *in vivo* interaction of mercury with sulphur), all types of chemical interaction are weak and readily reversible. Indeed, most ligands interact with their receptor sites in this rather 'loose' manner. This, in itself, emphasizes that the degree of precision of their geometrical matching is of paramount importance in the stabilization of their association.

Agonism versus antagonism

A receptor site pR is highly selective, in that its geometry severely restricts the number of potential ligands. For any given receptor site pR there may be one or more agonistic ligands pDa and one or more antagonistic or 'blocking' ligands pDb. An agonist initiates physiological events, whilst an antagonist inhibits or blocks the effect of an agonist. The effect of an antagonist pDb is only apparent when it diminishes the effect of either an endogenous or exogenous agonist pDa, e.g. part of a hormone or a drug, respectively.

Physicochemical concepts in agonism and antagonism

It has been suggested that, in the absence of a binding molecule D, each receptor molecule R oscillates between two subtle variations in shape – one (Ra) associated with agonism, the other (Rb) with antagonism (Katzung, 2001) – whilst, at the same time, the coarse geometry of pR is maintained. Furthermore, within any group of receptors, and in the absence of D, the concentration of the Ra form at any particular moment is presumed to be low. This, of course, implies that an unoccupied receptor must spend more time in the Rb than the Ra state.

It may be proposed that the subsequent docking of D at R results in the emergence of van der Waals' forces between various atoms of pD and pR (see below, *Van der Waals' forces and the Casimir effect*), and hence a steric stabilization of R and subsequent provocation of an appropriate response. That is to say, the oscillation between the two alternative molecular shapes of R ceases, with the adoption of a stable conformation (either Ra or Rb). Here, it will be maintained that the origin of the agonistic versus antagonistic conformation of the van der Waals' forces is in fact determined by the 'fine' geometry of the apposition of pD with pR, in contrast to the 'coarse' geometry of the lock and key mechanism described previously. The variables involved are the fine surface geometries of both pD and the receptor site pR.

As far as fine geometry is concerned, in the absence of pD, pR oscillates between two states: pRa (agonism) and pRb (antagonism). A ligand pDa, which behaves as an agonist, differs in fine geometry from a ligand pDb, which behaves as an antagonist – even where their coarse geometries are essentially similar. That is to say, their 'affinities' towards either pRa or pRb are different. However, in the case of a so-called 'partial agonist', whilst there may be a dominant affinity towards pRa, there is also a lesser affinity to pRb. Hence, for any given group of receptors occupied by a particular partially agonistic drug, the majority will be stabilized to the Ra conformation, and the minority to Rb. (It should also be noted that a specific receptor may produce different effects in different cells. Hence, a drug D which combines with a particular species of receptor R may be an agonist with regard to one type of cell and an antagonist with regard to another. That is to say, the Ra conformation for one cell functions as the Rb conformation for another. For example, tamoxifen acts as an agonist on oestrogen receptors in bony tissue, but as an antagonist on the oestrogen receptors of the breast. Additionally, there is 'functional antagonism', where different agonists bind with different types of receptor on the same cell, though with opposing physiological potentials, e.g. noradrenaline contracts the vascular smooth muscle cell, whilst acetylcholine relaxes it.)

Let us now examine the nature of the van der Waals' forces themselves in some detail.

Van der Waals' forces and the Casimir effect

Van der Waals' forces (VWF) are weak forces between atoms or molecules which diminish according to the sixth or seventh power of their distance of separation. Conventionally, they are viewed as an induced form of electrostatic attraction. In the field of general chemistry, they are the responsible for the lattice energy of molecular crystals. Our concern, however, is their relationship with biological receptor activity.

It has been suggested that VWF arise more fundamentally as a result of the **Casimir effect** (Puthoff, 1990; Haisch et al., 1997). This effect itself is seen under experimental conditions as a force of attraction between two uncharged flat metal plates which have been closely approximated. According to quantum mechanics, a vacuum is not empty, but full of energetic particles. Even when a molecule is cooled to absolute zero, apart from the energy it possesses because of its mass (in accordance with $E = mc^2$), there is still a considerable amount of other residual energy. This is said to result from the existence of an appropriately named **zero point field** (McTaggart, 2001). The Casimir effect is most simply explained by assuming that the two metal plates exclude virtual photons (from the zero point field) of wavelengths longer than their distance of separation. As a result, the photonic energy density between the plates is less than that on their outside surfaces. They are thus pushed together. A similar effect can be envisaged as occurring between molecules or atoms, giving rise to a weak form of attraction. In this respect, the electrostatic effect described in connection with VWF becomes a secondary phenomenon, rather than a primary one. (For those interested in such matters, it is also believed that the reason why the electron – which is negative – does not plunge into the atomic nucleus – which is positive – as might be expected from classical physics, is that it is supplied with energy from the zero point field. In this regard, the electron may be visualized as being enveloped by a cloud of virtual photons emanating from that field.)

Further experiments with regard to the Casimir effect have shown that the way in which it is manifest is highly sensitive to the geometry of the surfaces of the approximated plates, in terms of both their general contour and fine surface details (Mohideen and Roy, 1998). Indeed, under certain geometric circumstances, the **Casimir force** may even become repulsive – implying that the virtual photonic energy is then greater between the plates than outside them. We might further envisage that some form of Casimir effect occurs when pD interacts with pR, but its strength and direction of action (attraction or repulsion) will vary according to the fine geometry of the approximated surfaces. Furthermore, there is nothing to forbid one zone of such an approximation yielding a different manifestation of the Casimir force from another, though with a summational or nett attractive result. Neither is there anything to prevent this same force coexisting with ionic interaction or hydrogen bonding at the same site.

It is not unreasonable to propose that the Casimir effect which emerges from the juxtaposition of pD with pR forms part of a continuous electromagnetic field with the steric forces of bonding between the atoms of R. Thus, it may be proposed that the specific Casimir effect of that juxtaposition leads to specific stabilization of the shape of R. According to the exact nature of that effect, which depends on the fine geometry of pD and pR, so the result will be either agonism or antagonism (In the case of partial agonists, this affinity is less cut and dried. This probably results from a certain inaccuracy in geometrical matching, which itself enables subtle random variations in the docking position to occur. As a result of their influence on the Casimir effect, so most of these variations will be associated with agonism, and the remainder with antagonism.)

Furthermore, the closer the approximation of pD to pR, the stronger will be the overall Casimir force. Many molecular species of D exhibit the property of chirality (stereoisomerism), and exist as enantiomeric pairs. That is to say, they are either left- or right-handed, or mirror images of each other. For any given receptor pR, one enantiomer (left or right) will be more active than the other. Indeed, it is the geometry of pR which determines which of these two geometric entities will dock more closely. A stronger manifestation of the Casimir force results in greater agonistic or antagonistic effects.

Summation of geometric conformation

A useful way of conceptualizing the matching of pD with pR in general is to view them as mathematical sets (Lessell, 2002) indicative of their coarse geometry alone: {pD} and {pR}. The drug–receptor geometric complex that they form is thus {pD} + {pR}. Since pR has the negative geometry of pD, it follows that {pR} = {-pD}. Hence, {pD} + {pR} = {pD} + {-pD} = {0}; where {0} indicates an empty or null set. In other words, the functional geometry of the receptor site disappears – or the peg has filled the hole (see Figure 3.3). Obviously, if we were to examine the peg and hole microscopically, we would find small gaps. To fill those gaps we would need glue, which, in terms of our current theory, is provided by the virtual photons of the Casimir effect (Figure 3.3).

Substitution with the field concept

Although pD and pR are usually viewed as physical entities, it is perfectly legitimate to view them as 'fields'. As suggested by Einstein, matter itself is merely a condensed form of energy. We may thus consider pD and pR as fields (indicated by ★) composed of electromagnetic and other forms of energy (gravitational, thermal, etc.). Both pD★ and pR★ may be expressed as geometrical sets: {pD★} and {pR★} (more fully expressed as {pDa★} or {pDb★}, and {pRa★} or {pRb★}, respectively). In terms of coarse geometry, {pD★} + {pR★} = {0}. Of course, linking these two fields is the 'Casimir field', with its effect on receptor response (Figure 3.3).

Remedies as fields

Homeopathic remedies may be derived from either agonists or antagonists. A potentized homeopathic remedy F at a receptor site, being a biophotonically projected holographic image, may be considered as a subset F★ of E★, where E★ is the general electromagnetic field of the body, or that of *in vitro* cellular preparations (Lessell, 2002). However, this biophotonic image is extremely weak and devoid of any significant biological action in its own right, so it must be fortified by the incorporation of an additional type of

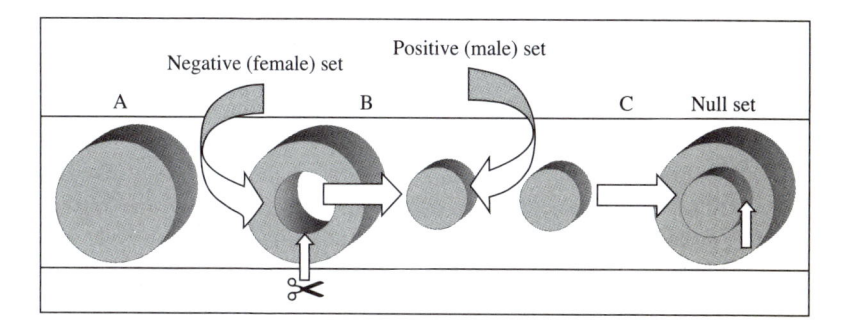

Figure 3.3
The basic coarse geometric principles involved in homeopathic pharmacodynamics and drug–receptor docking are simply illustrated by means of a block, as shown in **A**. **B** shows a cylindrical section being cut and removed from the block. The curved arrows indicate which cylinder represents a positive geometric set and which represents a negative one. In **C**, the positive set has been replaced within the negative, and the cut surfaces disappear, producing an empty or null set. The site of the Casimir effect/field, which acts as a thin layer of 'glue', is indicated by the vertical arrow.

electromagnetic energy from E★. As with ligands in general, usually only part of this fortified homeopathic field, i.e. pF★, will be of relevance to pR★.

pF★ corresponds geometrically to the whole or part of a single species of molecule or ion which has imprinted itself on the molecular memory of the diluent. It may be suggested, however, that the image of pF★ is not projected continuously, but intermittently. It may be envisaged that this arises because the fundamental hologram itself is only manifest intermittently (or in brief flashes, if you like). Intermittent projection implies the superimposition of pF★ on pR★ for only a few microseconds at a time – a period we shall call dt. In this respect pF★ is 'in competition' with the projection of the images of other molecules or ions that comprise F★, which also appear intermittently for the same brief period dt. Since they bear no appropriate geometrical relationship with pR★, they are devoid of any biological effect. All such projections at pR★ are exclusive, i.e. different types of image are not manifest at the same time.

Governed by the laws of probability, for any given period of time t seconds, the amount of that time $[\Sigma dt]_{pF\star}$ devoted to the intermittent manifestation of pF★ at the receptor site is actually related to the corresponding value of what we have termed $\Gamma\%$ (see Chapter 2, *Impurities*). As a result, where F★ is representative of two molecules X and Y, with $\Gamma\%$ values of 64% and 4% respectively (see Chapter 2, *Impurities*, Example 1), the theoretical ratio of $[\Sigma dt]_{pX\star}$ to $[\Sigma dt]_{pY\star}$ will be $[64/4]:1 = 16:1$. Since we are dealing with probability, the greater the value of t, the less the deviation from theoretical values of $[\Sigma dt]$ and any derivative ratios. Assuming, for the sake of argument, that pY rather than pX is in geometrical correspondence to pR, then for about 96% of the duration of the biological presence of the remedy field F★, pR★ will be 'occupied' by either the inappropriate pX★ (64%) or an amorphous image (32%). Hence, where t is taken to be 100 seconds, $[\Sigma dt]_{pY\star}$ will be in the region of 4 seconds. In this case, the chances of a significant physiological change being generated are slim. In this manner, molecules or ions that are poorly represented in molecular memory produce little or no biological response. Even where repeated potentization produces a 100% occupancy of molecular memory solely by the images of X (94.1 Γ%) and Y (5.9 Γ%), the value of $[\Sigma dt]_{pY\star}$, where t = 100 seconds, approximates to only 5.9 seconds. Of course, where the more significant pX is geometrically matched to pR, and thus pX★ to pR★, the situation is vastly more favourable.

Let us now consider E★ to be in the form of a geometric set {E★}, F★ to be a geometric subset {F★} of {E★}, and pF★ to be a geometric subset {pF★} of {F★}. As pF★ is a subset of F★, and thus of E★, so {pF★} is a subset of {E★}.

On occasion, {pF★} is of opposite coarse geometry to {pR★}, rather like {pD★}. Hence, {pF★} + {pR★} = {0} (see Figure 3.3). Again, the two are linked by a Casimir field. As might be expected, this produces a receptor effect similar to that of the interaction of a real ligand – be it pDa or pDb – with pR. Such effects are mainly seen with remedies derived from agonists, and usually in association with the following:

1. The prescription of very high potencies of decimal or centesimal remedies in chronic disease.
2. Too frequent repetition of remedies. } Often leading to aggravation
3. Persons prone to idiosyncratic homeopathic response (so-called 'sensitive' subjects).
4. *In vitro* experiments on cellular material (Ennis and Brown, 2001).
5. The prescription of hormonal remedies (e.g. *Secretin, FSH*).

Homeopathic blocking or shielding

More commonly, however, {pF★} has a similar coarse geometry to {pR★} – which, of course, is the negative of {pD★}. In other words, {pF★} = {pR★} in our restricted geometrical sense. Hence, {pF★} + {pR★} = {pR★} + {pR★} = 2{pR★}. This expresses the fact that we now have two similar surfaces at the same site, with {pF★} superimposed on, or shielding, {pR★}. Although no active physiological response is produced, there are other consequences. For example, {pF★} now blocks {pD★} by preventing its access to {pR★} (see Figure 3.4). Furthermore, where D is already closely attached to R, it will be displaced by the intervention of {pF★}. Such shielding, which affects both agonists and antagonists equally, is not dependent on the establishment of a Casimir field between {pF★} and {pD★}. Where a disease factor (e.g. a bacterial infection, a genetic programme) produces a toxin or excess of an autacoid T, which results in a disease pattern similar to the physiological effect of a drug D, it may be assumed that this follows from a similarity of part of its geometry {pT} to {pD}. It thus follows that {pF★}, which is pharmaceutically derived from D, can block the geometrical interaction of {pT★} with {pR★}. Where T is already attached to R, it will be displaced, and any further attachment will be blocked. As a result, the disease response tends to abate.

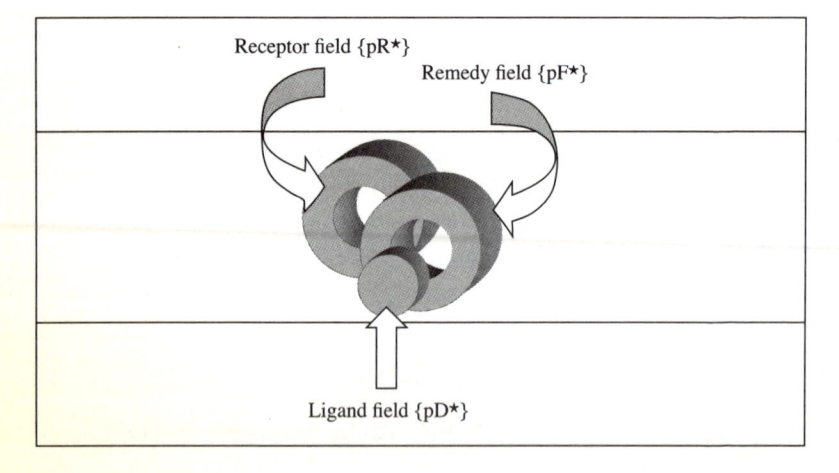

Figure 3.4
An abstract representation of homeopathic shielding using blocks. The arrows indicate the various fields involved. The ligand field is shielded from the receptor field by the remedy field.

Allergenic isopathy

We may consider that an allergic reaction is a cascade of events initiated by the interaction of an allergen J with a specific receptor site R. In this sense, J functions as an agonistic drug. One well known variety of R is the IgE protein attached to tissue mast cells and blood basophils. A potentized remedy derived from J, when manifest in a negative geometric form, can be used to block R against J. However, if manifest in its positive form, an aggravation of symptoms will occur. The circumstances under which this commonly occurs have been described in this chapter (see above, *Remedies as fields*).

The term **isopathy** is a general term which refers to the treatment of a disease by means of a remedy derived from the precipitating agent itself, be it a chemical substance, pollen, food allergen or micro-organism.

Viral remedies (viral nosodes)

Some important potentized remedies are made from material containing viruses (e.g. *Parotidinum* – the mumps nosode). Before a virus invades a cell, it docks at a surface receptor protein. It may be supposed that the effect of the appropriate remedy is to occupy the receptor site, and so deny the virus access to the cell. This will occur whether the remedy is either a positive or a negative geometrical image of the external contours of the virus. The occupancy of the receptor site by a positive remedy field does not lead, as with a virus, to the invasion of the cell.

Homeopathic blocking of therapeutic drugs

On the basis of this theory of Type I action, it might be envisaged that there will be instances where the efficacy of a therapeutic drug will be reduced by the blocking action of some homeopathic remedy. In fact, such occurrences are rare. For example, it is believed that the administration of homeopathic *Arnica* before giving a local anaesthetic will occasionally prevent the onset of satisfactory anaesthesia. More commonly, where a drug D, or a pathogenic autacoid or bacterial toxin T, is present in high concentrations in the tissue fluids, {pD★} or {pT★} penetrates the shield created by {pF★}, thereby gaining access to {pR★}. Some failures of homeopathic therapy result from this phenomenon, and measures must be introduced to reduce the levels of T. This is termed **detoxification**, and may be achieved in a number of different ways, homeopathically or otherwise. In homeopathy, the administration of so-called 'drainage' remedies to encourage the excretion or destruction of T via, for example, the liver and kidneys, may be suggested. In this respect, the activity of an enzyme Z involved in the degradation of T may be promoted by a potentized remedy of positive geometry derived from an agonist. Alternatively, where Z is inhibited by an antagonist, a remedy of negative geometry derived from either an agonist or antagonist will also promote this function.

Homeopathic action of material doses of drugs

Early in the history of homeopathy, it was customary for Hahnemann to administer material or 'crude' doses of drugs on a homeopathic basis, e.g. up to 3 grains of *Ignatia* (depending on age); $\frac{1}{5}-\frac{1}{2}$ grain of *Opium* (1 Nuremberg grain = 62mg) (Hahnemann, 1797: 1, 2). These significant doses were, however, quite small compared with allopathic usage of the same era. How could they have worked?

Let us suppose that an agonistic toxin or autacoid T causes a particular disease by occupancy of a receptor R. Let us say that the effects of this resemble those caused by the administration of an agonistic drug D to a healthy individual. Thus, D and T will dock at R in a similar manner – though, where D is either a partial agonist or binds less closely than T (i.e. with a lesser Casimir force), its biological effects will be less. T must now compete with the less aggressive D for R. This mechanism, which can be termed 'competitive agonism', depends on D being less toxic than T.

There is, however, a second mechanism, which may be more generally important. By giving material doses of D (but insufficient to cause overt toxicity), we effectively enhance the availability of ligands for R. As a result of this increased concentration of ligands, there then follow, after a possible initial aggravation of the disease symptomatology, receptor **desensitization** and **down-regulation**. These phenomena are associated with agonistic varieties of T and D. Desensitization is the generation of reduced receptor response over seconds or minutes. Once the agonist has been removed, full recovery often occurs within a quarter of an hour. However, of perhaps greater significance is down-regulation, a useful common example of which occurs in those addicted to chillies. After repeated exposure to capsaicin, the oral receptors become down-regulated, with progressive reduction of sensation and the demand for 'hotter and hotter' foods (from tikka to Thai, as one might say). Down-regulation is slower in onset (over hours or days) than desensitization but more prolonged and profound in its effect, involving such things as decrease in receptor biosynthesis, internalization of receptors to the cytoplasm of the cell, and also their actual degradation. As a result of these processes, the cure of the disease is accelerated.

It is important to note that very minute material quantities of drugs, as found residually in potentized remedies of dilution range 1 in 10^6–10^{24} or higher (Samal and Geckeler, 2001), are usually insufficient to result in the effects described above when given in their normal clinical dosage.

Duration of action of potentized remedies

It will be appreciated that {pF*}, being purely a subset of the general electromagnetic field of the body, is not subject to chemical locking. Thus, it cannot be unlocked either. Nor is it really undocked. A slightly simplified view would be that, like the old soldier, it merely fades away with the passage of time – minutes to days, according to circumstances. However, its disappearance is hastened by anything that causes a profound disturbance of the general electromagnetic field of the body. This occurs quite naturally in the course of acute illnesses (and less naturally, though perhaps more enjoyably, by consuming large amounts of strong coffee). Conversely, higher serial potencies are associated with molecular or ionic images of greater intensity, and this in itself tends to prolong the life of each dose; such an effect being disadvantageous if symptomatic aggravation occurs. Nevertheless, as with material drugs, the duration of biological effect is often governed by factors other than mere presence at the receptor site. In many instances, the cascade of physiological events which are initiated by receptor occupancy persist for some time after the remedy has faded away. In others, despite persistent receptor occupancy, the duration of action may be limited by the phenomena of receptor desensitization and down-regulation.

Explanation of the actions of *Arnica* and *Euphrasia*

The crude mother tincture of *Arnica montana* is often applied topically and effectively to limit traumatic bruising. Rather atypically, homeopathic potencies of *Arnica* of virtually any 'strength' (usually 6c–1M) usually produce the same effect when given by mouth. That is to say, the potentized remedy does not have the opposite effects of the crude drug, as is normally to be expected with remedies in general. It is true that crude *Arnica* administered by mouth may produce haemorrhages (Hughes and Dake, 1886), but this is a toxic reaction quite unconnected with its normal area of activity. Indeed, *Arnica* tincture should never be given by mouth for clinical purposes.

Let us assume that the crude tincture acts, at least in part, by inducing the constriction of capillaries and venules which have been dilated by an agonistic autacoid C, released at the time of trauma and subsequently. It will be further maintained that this is caused by some principal molecular component of *Arnica* which acts as an antagonist to C at the same receptor site, so reducing the degree of vasodilatation and bleeding into the tissues.

It is important to emphasize that a remedy of negative geometry produces blocking or shielding at the receptor site, and that a remedy of positive geometry derived from an antagonist will effectively do the same. Hence, the potentized remedy derived from *Arnica* tincture will also serve to block the action of the agonist C, whether it be geometrically positive or negative. In a sense, therefore, both the potentized and crude forms of *Arnica* act essentially as pharmacological antagonists with respect to C, with the development of similar physiological consequences.

The induction of haemorrhage by giving crude *Arnica* by mouth is probably a totally different phenomenon, involving the presence of other constituent molecules with only a weak ability to have such a deleterious effect on the blood vessels. This effect, either locally or systemically, will be thus unapparent with the small doses absorbed through the skin. The fact that these molecules do not manifest themselves significantly when given in potentized form can be simply explained in two ways. Firstly, if their relative concentration in the tincture is significantly less than that of the major antagonistic component, the relative presence of their geometry within the potentized remedy will be even smaller (see Chapter 2, *Impurities*). Secondly, assuming them to be agonists, when they present in a geometrically negative form – which is usually the case – they will actually block or shield their own receptor sites.

Euphrasia officinalis behaves in rather the same way in the treatment of acute conjunctivitis. The well-diluted, though unsuccussed, mother tincture may be applied topically, or the remedy may be given in a potentized form by mouth – with comparable results. The mechanism involved is probably similar to that involving *Arnica*, with *Euphrasia* manifesting antagonistic properties towards various agonistic inflammatory molecules. Moreover, giving crude *Euphrasia* by mouth may produce inflammation of the eye (Hughes and Dake, 1888) but, as with *Arnica*, this is probably due to the presence of molecules other than those which are normally involved in the clinical situation.

Explanation of the actions of *Mercurius* and *Arsenicum*

The toxic effects of mercury are mainly attributable to its ready ability to form covalent bonds with sulphur. In this respect, mercury interacts with the sulphydryl or thiol group –SH. Sulphydryl groups are to be found in many substances, including the common amino acid cysteine, and thus in proteins and polypeptides, including enzymes. With regard to receptors, in that the mercury–sulphur covalent bond is particularly strong, the coarse geometry of the site of interaction is less relevant than in the more usual case of a loosely bound drug. We might presume that many aspects of mercurial toxicity are due to what may be termed a 'non-specific action' on a variety of classes of receptor site, normally and specifically bound by various endogenous regulatory ligands; though with the proviso that each and every one contains the all important sulphydryl group.

Nevertheless, it might be suggested that the actual effect of mercury on the receptor macromolecule R, as with drugs in general, is to stabilize its conformation to the agonistic form Ra or, more commonly (especially with enzymes), to the antagonistic version Rb. In addition to the existence of a covalent bond between mercury and sulphur, there is a Casimir effect between atoms adjacent to that atom of sulphur and the mercury atom itself, the nature of which is determined by the fine geometry of that juxtaposition. It is presumably this effect, rather than the covalency, which selects the conformational outcome. As a result, homeopathically potentized mercury (*Mercurius*), though devoid of any ability to form covalent bonds with sulphur, may well influence receptor sites containing sulphydryl groups, thereby exerting a therapeutic effect in diseases with a similar symptomatology to that of mercurial poisoning. Furthermore, when administered in cases of mercurial toxicity, in either negative or positive geometric form, *Mercurius* may prevent the formation of new bonds between material mercury and sulphur at those sites. However, in view of the strength of established covalent bonds, it is less likely that it could actually displace mercury which is already bound.

Arsenic also exerts many, though not all, of its effects via a predilection for sulphydryl groups. On this basis, it may be thought that the symptomatic effects of arsenic poisoning should show some strikingly close similarities with those of mercury toxicity. This, however, is not the case. Thus, we might conceive that the initial attraction of either 'drug' to a particular sulphydryl group at a receptor site is due to the establishment of an appropriate and individualized Casimir effect. This, as previously stated, is determined by the fine geometry of the opposed surfaces of the drug and receptor. Should that effect be of appropriate distribution throughout the zone of juxtaposition, and of adequate strength, then the drug will be attracted to the receptor site and bound covalently. Should it be inappropriately distributed, weak, or even repulsive, then covalent bonding will not occur. In this way, each drug will possess its own range of compatible receptors. Likewise, the fields of their potentized forms, *Mercurius* and *Arsenicum*, will also be geometrically selective in their affinities, and thus their therapeutic effects.

Part Two
Non-receptor-mediated action of remedies (Type II action)

Fundamental ideas

There are certain homeopathic effects on the physiology and psyche which cannot be interpreted in terms of receptor mechanisms. Furthermore, where a potentized remedy is derived from a substance with a major constituent in the form of a physiological cation (such as Na^+ in salt), these effects cannot be interpreted in terms of a direct action on those mechanisms which identify and transport the material ion itself (e.g. Na^+/K^+ ATPase). (The same must apply to remedies derived from ions which act as 'substitutes' for physiological ions, such as Li^+.)

Although it must be suggested that non-receptor-mediated actions can occur with any potentized remedy, irrespective of derivation, their existence is perhaps best inferred from the properties of remedies containing significant geometrical correspondences to the important physiological cations of Na^+ (e.g. *Natrum muriaticum*), K^+ (e.g. *Kali phosphoricum*), Ca^{2+} (e.g. *Calcarea fluorica*) and Mg^{2+} (e.g. *Magnesia phosphorica*). Here, the main problem lies in the proposition that the potentized remedy expresses the true surface geometry of the ion (negative or positive), but lacks any expression of charge. Since the matter of charge is of great importance in the way these ions are processed in the physiology, it follows that their homeopathic derivatives are unlikely to be handled by the same mechanisms. However, on clinical grounds it would seem that *Natrum muriaticum*, for example, controls the distribution of Na$^+$ (and thus water) within the compartments of the body, and that *Magnesia phosphorica* exerts a subtle influence on Mg^{2+} levels. This is inferred, albeit tenuously, from the use of *Natrum muriaticum* to control benign fluid retention and depression (compare lithium), and the use of *Magnesia phosphorica* in the prevention or treatment of simple cramps (since low Mg^{2+} levels predispose to cramping). It might, therefore, be proposed that the mode of action of such ionic remedies on the Na$^+$ and Mg^{2+} regulatory mechanisms is of an indirect nature. The possible reabsorption of Mg^{2+} via the renal tubules, for example, should not be due to any direct effect of the remedy on the kidneys.

Further concepts of disease

In Part One of this chapter, we visualized disease in terms of a pathogenic autacoid or toxin T interacting either agonistically or antagonistically with a receptor macromolecule R. In reality, of course, there may be several species of T interacting with several geometrically compatible species of R at one and the same time. However, as a consequence of this effect and others (e.g. psychology, organ failure, hypoxia, dehydration, nutritional deficiency), in both acute and chronic diseases the physiology becomes disturbed. This results in a corresponding disturbance of the general electromagnetic field E★ of the body. Since E★ is in a state of balance with the physiology, it follows that anything which will correct E★ will also tend to rectify any associated physiological disturbance. The relationship between the general electromagnetic field, the pathophysiology and the symptomatology may be expressed thus:

$$[E\star \leftrightarrow \text{Pathophysiology}] \rightarrow \text{Symptoms}$$

So, when a remedy F acts at a receptor site R allocated to T, it may be said that it treats the pathophysiology *directly*. Conversely, when it acts on the disturbance of E★ caused by the interaction of R and T or by other factors, it treats the pathophysiology *indirectly*. It should be appreciated, however, that correction of the physiology by either method is sometimes unachievable unless certain other important indicated measures are also carried out, such as nutritional correction and rehydration. Furthermore, whilst these proximal Type I and II actions of remedies may be swift, actual clinical improvement in chronic disease may take some considerable time (weeks to months). In contrast, the response in acute disease is often rapid (minutes to days).

Geometric concepts

It may be suggested that one of the normal aspects of E★ is the formation of three-dimensional patterns in its magnetic component (by particular orientations of its particles). In association with a state of disease, it may be proposed that this pattern is corrupted. Such a disturbance may be generalized or localized to the region of particular dysfunctional organs, and may be considered as a non-geometric subset of E★, namely pE★. Furthermore, part of a homeopathic remedy field pF★ can be considered as a magnetic holographic interference pattern in its own right within E★, but, in contrast to Type I actions, without biophotonic projection. As such, pF★ and pE★ may interact directly. In this respect, following the lines discussed in Part One (see above, *Remedies as fields*), it is useful to assume that pF★ is representative of the whole or part of a single molecule or ion, and that it is manifest intermittently, and in 'probabilistic competition' with the other components of the F★ hologram, according to their corresponding $\Gamma\%$ values. The greater the value of $[\Sigma dt]_{pF\star}$ for any given period of time t seconds, the greater the influence on pE★.

We may interpret the interaction of the magnetic pattern of pF★ with that of pE★ in terms of a set geometry. For, although there is no overt geometrical interaction along the lines suggested for Type I actions, nor any interposed Casimir field, the interaction of the magnetic patterns may be conceptualized more easily by ascribing to it similar geometrical rules. In other words, we shall

Table 3.1
The symptomatic consequences of the geometric status of $\{pE^\star\}$

Geometric Status	Level of Symptoms
$\{pE^\star\}$	Characteristic →
$\{0^\star\}$	Diminishing ↓
$2\{pE^\star\}$	Aggravated ↑

imagine that both $pF^\star$ and $pE^\star$ exist in projected geometrical forms.

Therefore, in considering $E^\star$ to be a geometric set $\{E^\star\}$, we shall now regard the electromagnetic component of a disease as a geometric subset of $\{E^\star\}$, namely $\{pE^\star\}$. It follows that this may be eliminated by a field of opposite geometrical configuration $\{pF^\star\}$ produced by the administration of an appropriate homeopathic remedy F.

When $\{pF^\star\} = \{-pE^\star\}$, then $\{pE^\star\} + \{pF^\star\} = \{0^\star\}$; where $\{0^\star\}$ is an empty or null subset denoting the absence of field disturbance. This is a common state of affairs, and usually arises when $\{pF^\star\}$ is of negative geometry and $\{pE^\star\}$ is of positive configuration, though sometimes the reverse applies (see Figure 3.5). Either interaction tends to improve the physiology (see Table 3.1).

However, and less often, $\{pF^\star\} = \{pE^\star\}$. We then have $\{pE^\star\} + \{pF^\star\} = 2\{pE^\star\}$. This can also occur in two different theoretical ways, i.e. where both $\{pF^\star\}$ and $\{pE^\star\}$ are either geometrically positive or negative (see Figure 3.5). In either case, this essentially means that the partial disturbance of $E^\star$ is magnified. As a consequence, the corresponding physiological disturbance and its associated symptoms are also magnified (see Table 3.1). This occurs in the same clinical and *in vitro* situations as listed above in *Remedies as fields*. As a general rule, any aggravation of the disease and its symptoms is not of sufficient intensity to warrant concern, provided that no further doses of the remedy are given until that aggravation is no longer apparent. It is also true that, in many instances, aggravation is followed by physiological and symptomatic improvement. That is to say, the geometric polarity of {pF★} presumably becomes reversed, so as to cause {pE★} to become {0★}. A similar situation of 'geometric polarity reversal' may also occur in relation to aggravation produced by a receptor-mediated Type I action. Aggravations of any sort, whether followed by polarity reversal or

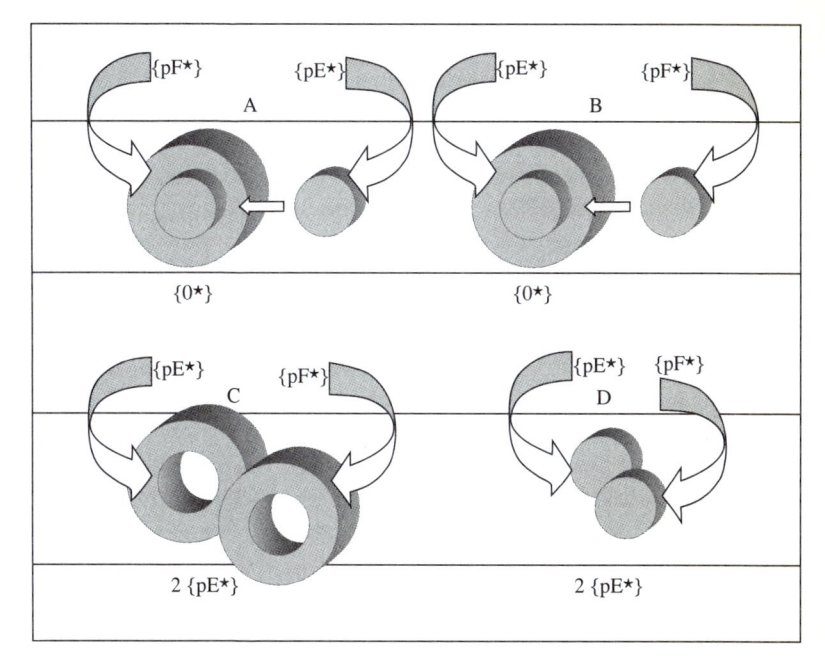

Figure 3.5
An abstract representation of the four basic theoretical geometrical interactions of a remedy field {pF★} with a subset {pE★} using blocks. **A** and **B** illustrate two alternative ways of forming a null subset {0★}. **C** and **D** illustrate two alternative ways of producing 2{pE★}. The hollow cylinders represent a negative geometric conformation, and the solid cylinders a positive one.

not, are more common in the treatment of chronic rather than acute disease.

Multiple subsets in chronic disease

In actual practice, physiological disturbances in chronic diseases are seldom treatable with single remedies; and the same occasionally applies to those of a more acute nature. This is because the aberrant geometric configuration of E★ can be highly complex. As a result, a number of different remedies must be applied (often sequentially) to cover the case. We may thus conceptualize that such a disturbance of E★ is composed of multiple geometric subsets: {^{1}pE★}, {^{2}pE★}, {^{3}pE★}, etc. Some remedies may only correspond to one subset, whilst others may cover two or more. Sometimes, whilst a well-chosen remedy manifests the opposite geometric field pattern of several subsets of E★, it also presents similar geometric patterns with regard to other such subsets. Thus, some symptoms remit, whilst others become aggravated. In many instances, it is then better to select a totally new remedy. In some cases, aggravation of symptoms may also be produced by a concomitant effect at the receptor level (Type I action).

In the case of a single remedy, the ability to target directly a number of different subsets depends in part on the number of different ions or molecules present in the original substance (tincture, etc.) which achieve significant geometric representation within the potentized product (see Chapter 2, *Impurities*). Complex mixtures of various potentized substances can also affect multiple subsets in a similar direct manner. There is also the matter of the chemical structure of each molecule, since those with a greater number of potential ligands have, when potentized, a greater potential to target several or many subsets. The same principles hold for Type I actions, where a variety of different species of receptor may be influenced by either a single or complex (i.e. mixed) prescription (see Chapter 4, *Complex prescriptions*).

Despite this description, there are some very simple geometries that may produce profound general physiological effects. These are exemplified by the polychrests (remedies of many uses) *Sulphur* and

Phosphorus. Here, we might propose that $\{^2pE^\star\}$, $\{^3pE^\star\}$, etc. depend strongly for their existence on $\{^1pE^\star\}$. Hence, when a polychrest of simple geometry directly eliminates that of the fundamental subset $\{^1pE^\star\}$, the other subsets, irrespective of their geometric complexity, are indirectly removed in consequence. This is rather like toppling a chimney stack by knocking out its bottom bricks.

The proposition that the geometry of a subset might sometimes be very simple, is also exemplified by theoretical disturbances of $E^\star$ which might characterize an excess or deficiency of a physiological cation. In this respect, let us suppose that, as a result of a disease X, there is a retention of Na^+. In that case, the geometry of the corresponding subset $\{^{Na^+}pE^\star\}$ will be representative, rather alchemically, of the superficial geometry of Na^+ itself. Furthermore, we shall make the assumption that its geometric form is positive. Hence, when a sodium remedy field $\{^{Na^+}pF^\star\}$ of negative geometric configuration is applied, via the administration of one of the *Natrum* (sodium) group of remedies, then $\{^{Na^+}pE^\star\}$ + $\{^{Na^+}pF^\star\} = \{0^\star\}$, and aggravation does not follow. With regard to the assumption that $\{^{Na^+}pE^\star\}$ is of positive geometry, it is likely that both physiological excesses and deficiencies of ions normally register in this manner. In this way, the ionic control mechanisms are merely 'instructed' to correct themselves, rather than being 'told' to act in any particular direction. The evidence – albeit slim and highly speculative – in support of this notion is that the *Magnesium* remedy field $\{^{Mg^{2+}}pF^\star\}$, which on theoretical grounds should normally be of negative geometric conformation, usually appears to treat states of mild Mg^{2+} deficiency without aggravation of symptoms, i.e. cramps. Were the subset $\{^{Mg^{2+}}pE^\star\}$ routinely of negative geometry in such cases, then aggravation would probably occur in most cases, since $\{^{Mg^{2+}}pE^\star\} + \{^{Mg^{2+}}pF^\star\} = 2\{^{Mg^{2+}}pE^\star\}$.

Returning now to disease X, this will be represented *in toto* by $\{^{Na^+}pE^\star\}$ plus one or more other subsets of $E^\star$. Hence, the reduction of $\{^{Na^+}pE^\star\}$ alone to the null subset $\{0^\star\}$ will probably result in only a trivial and temporary effect. Unless the remaining subsets are dealt with, the pathophysiology cannot revert to normal.

Sometimes physiological normalization is achievable by using a remedy derived from one particular sodium compound, where the complementary anion (CO_3^{2-}, SO_4^{2-}, etc.) provides the requisite effect on those subsets. At other times this must be supplied by a totally different type of remedy, such as one derived from a plant tincture or another mineral. Indeed, on the basis of the 'toppling chimney' analogy (see above), the subset $\{^{Na+}pE\star\}$ may not require any direct attack at all. Moreover, in many instances, it may well be by a combination of both Type I and Type II actions that the remedy achieves the therapeutic goal determined by the clinician.

Intermediate states

The geometrical analogy so far described, though practical, has its limitations. In terms of set geometry, $\{pF\star\}$ is sometimes neither the full negative nor the full positive of $\{pE\star\}$. That is to say, it produces intermediate results of enhancement or elimination of $\{pE\star\}$. In real terms, this means that the pattern of pF$\star$ does not exactly match that of pE$\star$. Therefore, what has been stated so far really only applies to well-chosen remedies with an exact positive or negative correspondence of pF$\star$ to pE$\star$. In other cases, short of a gross mismatch, we must expect either partial elimination of pE$\star$ or, less commonly, its partial enhancement.

There is also the matter of 'potency', which can be equated with 'intensity' or 'strength' of the magnetic field of pF$\star$. Although not stated previously as such, we have assumed that the magnetic fields pE$\star$ and pF$\star$ are of equal strength. However, where pF$\star$ is weaker than pE$\star$ and is also its negative, only partial correction can be produced. As a result, the prescription of a higher potency is usually warranted. In contrast, where pF$\star$ is stronger than pE$\star$ and is also its negative, then 'inversion' will occur, where pF$\star$ manifests itself in the place of pE$\star$. Thus, if we give too high a potency of *Silicea* to correct 'chilliness', we might find that the patient feels excessively hot. In consequence, no further doses of the remedy should be given until this problem has abated. Thereafter, if the symptom of chilliness returns, *Silicea* may be administered again, but in a lower potency.

The fact that different varieties of pF★ can interact with any given disturbance pEᴬ, albeit to different degrees, is of some clinical advantage, since it enables the practitioner to produce desirable effects with a range of remedies, rather than one in particular – the so-called 'simillimum' (see Chapter 1, *What is the 'simillimum'?*; *What is a 'similior'?*) – and with a variety of potencies (see Chapter 4, *Potency and therapeutic response*; *Dose repetition*). Indeed, were this not the case, failures of therapy would be more the rule than the exception.

Electromagnetic radiation remedies

There are a number of potentized remedies in homeopathy prepared from vials of alcohol–water which have been exposed to various types of electromagnetic phenomena for varying lengths of time. These include such remedies as *Sol* (sunlight), *VDU* and *Magnetis polus australis* (South pole of the magnet). It must be assumed that these only exhibit Type II actions, since any correspondence with specific receptors would seem unlikely. The possible ways in which they might be imprinted on the diluent have been discussed previously (see Chapter 2, *Electromagnetic energization*). Since waves are symmetrical about their horizontal axes, they have no morphological opposite – and their magnetic fields are similar in this respect. The properties of homeopathic positivity and negativity are probably only developed *in vivo*. This may entail the establishment of some form of chiral orientation of the magnetic particles of their fields (F★), so that one form is the mirror image of the other. Again, positive and negative geometric sets can be used to represent these opposite versions.

Conclusion

It is proposed that any given homeopathic remedy in any given biological situation may be associated with one or more Type I or Type II actions, or a combination of these, either simultaneously or in various sequences. Without the profound advances made in the last decade in the understanding of both the Casimir effect and receptor pharmacology, no comprehensive theory of Type I action would have been possible. In fact, without such collateral progress, any reasonable explanation of the mechanisms involved in the Similia Principle might have been beyond our reach. The former inability to explain the pharmacodynamics of homeopathy has been one of the greatest stumbling blocks to its general acceptance, despite the positive results of many properly conducted investigations.

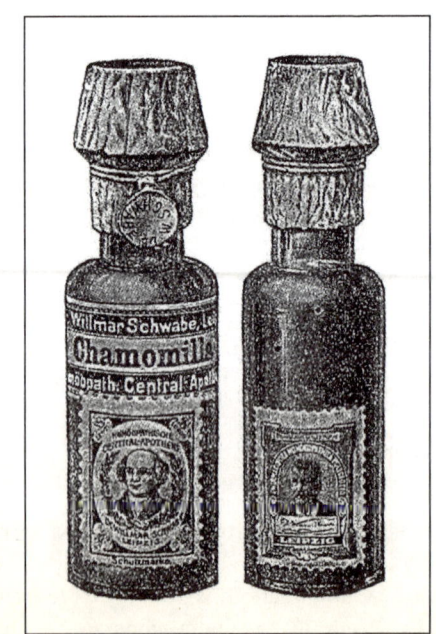

Figure 3.6
Bottles of homeopathic *Chamomilla* for domestic use. Elaborate by modern minimalist standards. Dr Willmar Schwabe Pharmacy, Leipzig, c. 1900.

One particular adverse effect to watch out for is associated with concurrent orthodox or herbal treatment, but is not due to any interaction between the remedy and the other medicine. It simply arises when the patient's condition improves as a result of homeopathy, in which case the dose of the orthodox or herbal medicine becomes too large and may require reduction.

4
Thinking about dosage and related matters

Introduction

In this chapter, we mainly examine the principles of dosage, i.e. the ways in which remedies may be administered, in what amounts, and with what precautions. A few additional tips on storage will also be given. Luckily for the busy clinician and retail pharmacist, who are largely concerned with fairly straightforward and basic prescriptions, there are a number of good books around which simplify the matters of both remedy selection and dosage. *The Complementary Formulary* (Lessell, 2001), for example, has been specifically designed for this purpose and is a most valuable asset where time allows for only brief consultation (even over the telephone).

In orthodox pharmacy, of course, the dosage of oral medication is a relatively simple matter of determining the amount required in milligrams in relation to weight or age, and when it should be taken. In homeopathic pharmacy, however, things are a little different. Here, the idea of dosage encompasses the following concepts:

1. The numerical potency of the remedy, e.g. 30c, D12, LM2. In each scale of serial dilution, a higher potency may be regarded as being of greater intensity than a lower, and having a lesser content of unintelligible geometric information (see Chapter 2, *Impurities*, Example 1). The following definitions are useful, albeit somewhat arbitrary. (The term 'attenuation' will be found in older books.)
   a. *Low* potency/attenuation: < 12c; <D12.
   b. *Medium* potency/attenuation: 12c–30c; D12–D30; LM1.
   c. *High* potency/attenuation: > 30c; >D30; LM2–LM30.
2. The means by which it is delivered, e.g. drops, tablets, pillules (see Table 4.1).
3. The material amount to be given, e.g. 1 drop, 1 pillule, 1 tablet.
4. The mode of administration, i.e. straight on the tongue or dispersed in a stated amount of water. If dispersed in water, whether all should be taken as a dose or some smaller quantity (e.g. 5ml). LM potencies are usually given in water; c and D potencies usually directly in solid form.

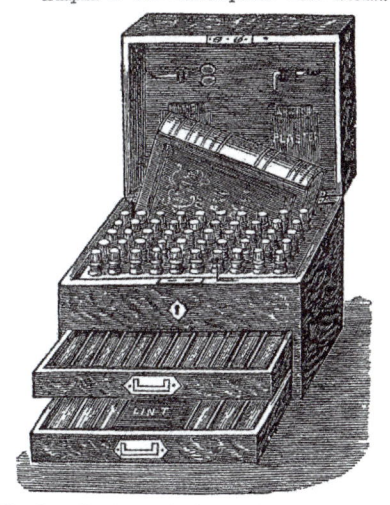

Figure 4.1
English advertisement for homeopathic remedies, 1875. From the *British Homoeopathic Medical and Pharmaceutical Directory* (London, Homoeopathic Publishing Co.).

5. Where administered in water, whether further succussion or dilution plus succussion is required as treatment progresses in order to increase the level of potency (so-called 'plussing').
6. The frequency of repetition – which is variable and flexible (see below, *Dose repetition*).

Except for reasons of safety and convenience, the age of the patient may be disregarded as far as dosage is concerned. Obviously a small infant should not be given a tablet without first crushing it. The weight of the patient can be similarly disregarded.

Mother tinctures

Most mother tinctures in homeopathic pharmacy are reserved for potentization. However, some are used topically, either diluted or undiluted. In diluted form they appear as lotions, creams, ointments, suppositories and eye drops. The occasional allergic reaction is, of course, to be expected. A few are administered by mouth (e.g. *Urtica*, *Crataegus*), usually in water, and it is important to check for possible adverse interactions with any concurrent orthodox or herbal medication (Lessell, 2001).

Mother tinctures should be stored in tightly stoppered bottles in a cool and dark area, but for no longer than 2 years from the date of manufacture. Glass is preferable to plastic, and neutral glass is preferable to soda glass. Some mother tinctures are prone to loss of solute by sedimentation. Should this occur, it is wise, in the interests of standardization, to avoid subjecting them to potentization, even though they may be perfectly satisfactory for other purposes.

Liquid potencies

The product of liquid phase potentization is termed a **liquid potency**. Each such product must be labelled correctly – e.g. *Euphrasia* 6c – since there is no standard or reliable method of assay for unlabelled potentized material. There are various avant-garde methods (e.g. pendulum dowsing), but these are hardly of any commercial value.

It is important to store liquid potencies in tightly stoppered vials, preferably of neutral glass and amber in colour. Large amounts, however, may be kept in 316-grade stainless steel containers with sprung lids and silicone-rubber seals. These have the advantages of durability, opacity and relative cheapness.

Liquid potencies must be protected from ultraviolet light and intense magnetic fields. As a liquid remedy ages, it slowly loses energy from its molecular memory. However, occasional agitation, as infrequently as once a month, preserves the level of information imprinted on the diluent.

Occasionally, liquid potencies are applied topically (e.g. *Graphites* D8 cream). Mostly, however, they are destined for systemic use. Some are available in sterile injectable form (e.g. *Ruta* for musculoskeletal problems), but more usually they are given orally in a variety of ways:

1. *Directly on the tongue.* For this purpose, the liquid potency should have an alcohol content of about 30%.
2. *In water.* The exact amount of water and the number of drops suggested will vary between practitioners. This method is particularly suitable for veterinary work with commercial animals, where the liquid potency is put in a trough or the like. In this regard, 4ml of liquid potency will effectively medicate about 455 litres of drinking water. This is a simple dilution of 1 in 1.138×10^5. In fact, it is probably unwise to exceed a simple dilution level of 1 in 4.125×10^5 (Lessell, 1994).
3. *As a medicated solid form.* For the purpose of medicating solids, the alcohol content of the liquid potency should ideally be in the range of 90–96%. Otherwise, the solid – which is composed of one or more sugars – becomes excessively sticky. Usually 1 or 2 drops per 10g suffices. This may be achieved manually for small quantities or mechanically (in rotating drums) for large amounts. The various solids that may be medicated, together with some useful notes, are given in Table 4.1.

Table 4.1
Solid dose media for liquid potencies

Solid dose form	Shape No. per gram Size	Major sugar	Minor sugar	Comments
Pillules/Pills ('granules' in non-Anglophone countries)	Spherical. 23/g (average)	Sucrose	**Lactose**	*Easily recognizable as homeopathic.* Most popular solid form. Unsuitable for vegans. Available in different sizes.
Granules(UK)/ Globules/ Globuli	Spherical. 350/g (average) Like poppy seeds.	**Lactose**	Sucrose	Convenient for travel kits. Convenient for doctor's bag. Difficult to handle. Unsuitable for vegans. Useful for infants. Useful in veterinary homeopathy. Essential for LM production (1600/g).
Tablets	Flat, round. Approximate diameter: 6mm	**Lactose**	Sucrose	*Confusion with orthodox tablets.* Unsuitable for vegans.
Crystals	= Granulated cane sugar.	Sucrose	–	Suitable for babies. Suitable for vegans. Dissolve easily in water. Confusion with plain sugar.
Powders	Very fine. Usually in folded paper packets.	**Lactose**	–	Time consuming to prepare. Unsuitable for vegans. *May be mistaken for narcotics.*

Dosage of liquid and solid forms

Usually only the most minute amount of liquid potency is required to produce a clinical effect. This is because the amplification zones of the mouth, oropharynx and elsewhere (see Chapter 3, *Introduction*) will sufficiently enhance the remedy after administration. Even the amount contained in a single granule is quite adequate to induce a response, and giving any more than the minimum does not generally increase the response. Hence, the easiest approach to dosage is to think of the number '1': 1 drop, 1 pillule, 1 granule, or 1 small pinch of crystals or powder. It is true that some manufacturers suggest larger doses than these – such as 2 pillules rather than 1, or whole tubes of granules in one go – which is obviously of some commercial advantage. Though this would seem to be an unnecessary extravagance, it is also true to say that a minority of individuals are sufficiently insensitive to warrant such doses. This perhaps arises from a relative insensitivity of their amplification sites. In consequence, there may be some justification in prescribing, e.g. 2 pillules rather than 1. Nevertheless, such people will usually obtain some benefit from the smallest material dose, and only differ from others by gaining an increased response from greater amounts.

There are also some very sensitive individuals who require less than 1 drop, 1 pillule, 1 granule, etc. In such people, these normal doses regularly give rise to either aggravated or new symptoms (see below, *Adverse effects of potentized remedies*). When this happens, a smaller material dose must be given. Technically, it is quite difficult to cut pillules or granules in half. However, a single pillule is easily crushed with the handle of a knife and dissolved in a wineglass of lukewarm water, thus creating a so-called 'wet dose' from a 'dry dose'. The patient may then be instructed to drink only half a glass of the resultant solution. Using a single drop in water is probably easier. However, since the remedy will adhere to the glass, irrespective of which method is used, it should be put through a standard high temperature cycle in a dishwasher primed with detergent, or left in sunlight for a few days after initial rinsing. The knife used for crushing should be treated similarly, and the person

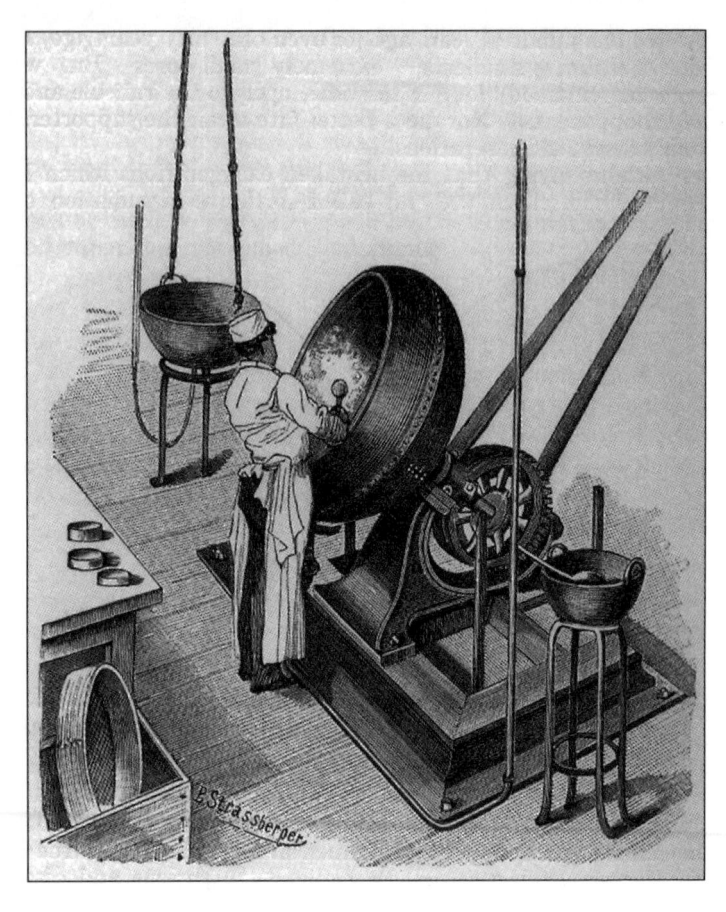

Figure 4.2
Manufacture of globules and pillules. German illustration, *c.* 1920. These are built up in layers by adding successive aliquots of syrup to the revolving drum.

administering the remedy should wash their hands thoroughly afterwards, scrubbing them with soap and hot water.

Beware of prescribing solid forms in patients with disaccharide intolerance. Lactose intolerance is more common than sucrose intolerance. People with 'cow's milk allergy' are intolerant of cow's milk protein (mainly casein), but usually tolerate lactose well. Alcoholics on Antabuse therapy should not be given the smallest amounts of alcohol, and liquid potencies for them must contain water alone. The same applies to certain religious groups. Bach Flower Remedies are also to be regarded as alcohol-based liquid potencies. The suggested dose is usually 2–4 drops (often in water). For chronic or subacute psychological syndromes, this amount is often given 3 or 4 times daily.

LM potencies are generally administered 'wet', by first dissolving a single granule/globule in purified water. Thereafter, however, considerable variations exist in the instructions issued by different practitioners as to dosage.

Triturated material

Where insoluble substances (e.g. sulphur) are intended for use in potencies up to 3c or D6, the triturated material, which is largely lactose, may be dispensed as such (i.e. in powder form), but is more usually compressed into flat tablets. The principles of dosage and storage are as for other solid forms. Some manufacturers, however, suggest that 2–4 tablets (according to the patient's age) constitute a dose. Again, there is no harm done by giving more than 1 tablet, and perhaps some good is done in the case of a homeopathically insensitive patient.

The so-called Biochemic Tissue Salts are essentially decimal scale homeopathic mineral remedies prepared in this manner, despite claims by their originator, Wilhelm Schüssler MD, that they were to be regarded as something different – this solely to establish a unique brand-name. Currently prepared on a large scale commercially, trituration is accomplished in porcelain mills.

Potency and therapeutic response

It is convenient to regard the theoretical intensity (or **functional therapeutic potency**) of a geometric imprint on a diluent as conforming to a scale with a range of 0 (minimum) to 5 (maximum) in arbitrary units – perhaps best visualized as graduated shades of grey (see Table 4.2). However, the relationship between this theoretical intensity and the numerical level of potency on any particular scale of serial dilution is not linear. Table 4.2 illustrates the approximate relationship between the potencies in regular use and the theoretical intensity. Moreover, the therapeutic effect may be regarded as being related to the level of intensity, with a maximal response corresponding to level 5 in people of average sensitivity to homeopathic treatment. Whilst the therapeutic effect generally increases with intensity, so does the risk of aggravation of symptoms (see below, *Adverse effects of potentized remedies*). In persons of great sensitivity, a maximal response may be achieved at a level of intensity even as low as 1, with the prescription of higher potencies causing no increase in therapeutic effect, but only uncomfortable aggravation.

Dose repetition

Dose repetition varies according to the following factors:

1. *The potency of the remedy.* For any given situation, a low potency (e.g. 6c) requires more frequent repetition than a medium (e.g. 30c), and a medium more frequent repetition than a high (e.g. 200c).
2. *Whether the disease or syndrome is acute or chronic.* Acute diseases may require the prescription of either low or medium (or occasionally high) potencies quite frequently, e.g. 6c or 30c, 3 or 4 times daily. Chronic diseases are sometimes treated with low or medium potencies once or twice daily, or with high potencies more cautiously, e.g. 200c, 1 dose twice weekly. Very acute situations, such as shock or croup, may require

Table 4.2
The approximate relationship between intensity and numerical potency according to scale

Intensity (Functional therapeutic potency)	Numerical potency according to scale		
	Centesimal scale	LM scale	Decimal scale
5 (max)	CM	LM30	–
4	1M	LM3	–
3	200c	LM2	–
<3, >2	100c	–	–
2	30c	LM1	D30
<2, >1	12c	–	D12
1	6c	–	D6
<1, >0	<6c	–	<D6
0 (min)	unpotentized substance		

repetition of a medium or high potency of a remedy every 10 minutes or so.

3. *The nature of the remedy.* Remedies derived from viruses or bacteria (or their toxins) – i.e. 'nosodes' – are given in medium or high potencies, but relatively infrequently in the treatment of chronic disease, e.g. once weekly. However, when used in acute disease (e.g. *Medorrhinum* for acute otitis media), much more frequent repetition is indicated, but the total number of doses given should be limited.
4. *The sensitivity of the patient.* Patients prone to either aggravations or swift responses with homeopathic remedies in general require less frequent dose repetition, and remedies of low potency.
5. *The response.* As the patient improves, so the frequency of repetition should be reduced, and the remedy eventually discontinued (see also Chapter 1, *Potencies and frequency of repetition*).

Storage of solid forms

For long-term storage, amber neutral glass vials are preferable. Plastic is only suitable for storage of up to 1 year or so, and goose quills, as used in the first quarter of the nineteenth century (when glass vials were scarce) have long since been abandoned. Once a liquid potency has been incorporated in a solid form, it becomes extremely stable, and will remain active for many decades – provided, of course, it is kept in a well-stoppered neutral glass vial, and away from sunlight and intense magnetic fields. Although any agitation of the pillules etc. will not produce any enhancement of molecular memory, neither does a liquid potency so stabilized in sugar tend to lose energy at any great rate. This stabilization is probably achieved by the transfer of imprinted information, though without intensification (increase in potency), from the liquid potency to sugar molecules, and, in the case of lactose, to water of crystallization. Thus, even a medicated solid form which has lost all or most of its free water and alcohol molecules may remain therapeutically effective for many years. Indeed, the purpose of ensuring that the stopper is tight is more to prevent unwanted exogenous contaminants entering than to limit the escape of water and alcohol. These contaminants are such things as water vapour from humid atmospheres (which makes the solids become sticky), bacteria and perfumes (see below, *Precautions in taking remedies*).

Precautions in taking remedies

The precautions in taking remedies are really very few:

1. The remedy is best dissolved on the tongue, or, if dispersed in water, then it should be held in the mouth for a few seconds before being swallowed.
2. Solid remedies should be handled minimally, and no aromatic substances (especially perfumes) should be present on the hands or fingers. It is likely that aromatic substances may adversely effect the informational amplification sites related to the mouth, nose and pharynx, and that at least

some of these are associated with the taste buds, and perhaps others with the olfactory receptors.
3. No food, drink or tooth-cleaning for 5 minutes either way of taking a remedy. Again, this is to prevent interference with the amplification sites. Peppermint is said to be the worst offender in this respect, but even onions and garlic have been quoted as being almost equally bad. Nevertheless, provided the 5-minute rule is observed, none of these things seems to be significantly problematical.
4. Coffee should be avoided, since it can be antidotal in some cases. This effect may be attributed to the production of a general disturbance of the electromagnetic field of the body (see Chapter 3, *Duration of action of potentized remedies*).

Adverse effects of potentized remedies

There is seldom, if ever, any adverse interaction of homeopathic remedies with orthodox medication, herbal prescriptions or nutritional substances. *Arnica* may be an exception, when taken prior to local anaesthesia (see Chapter 3, *Homeopathic blocking of therapeutic drugs*). However, there are occasionally adverse interactions with other potentized remedies being taken concurrently. Such interactions are classified as antidotal and inimical. Some of these are well documented (Gibson Miller, 2002).

The remedy *Silicea* should not be given to patients who have recently had any form of transplant or implant, since it favours the expulsion of foreign bodies which have incurred a rejection response. Shrapnel is another problem, as are other embedded projectiles, for in moving, such bodies may damage vital structures, e.g. the spinal cord. Dental fillings are, however, quite immune to this process, being no more than simple prostheses.

Perhaps the most common adverse effect is aggravation of symptomatology due to the prescription of a well-indicated remedy, but in too high a potency. This is mainly seen in the treatment of chronic rather than acute disease. It is said to occur less commonly with LM potencies, but these are not currently in general use for OTC purposes. Nevertheless, the reckless prescription of aggressive constitutional treatment in persons of grossly weakened physiology by over-enthusiastic practitioners can be a real problem (see Chapter 1, *Constitutional prescribing*).

In sensitive subjects, new and hitherto absent symptoms are occasionally experienced which are characteristic of the general properties of the remedy, rather than of the illness or of a constitutional predisposition. Such a symptom is often readily identified by consulting standard works on homeopathic materia medica, and is termed 'a proving' (or, more correctly, 'a clinical or sporadic proving'), whilst the patient is said 'to have proven the remedy'. Sometimes, even in subjects of average sensitivity, apparently new symptoms are, in fact, old ones which have recurred (see Chapter 1, *What is 'Hering's Law'?*). In both instances, the remedy should be discontinued, and further professional advice sought by those less experienced. If, however, a new symptom is neither a proving nor an old symptom in disguise, then it must be assumed, quite reasonably, that it has arisen through no fault of homeopathy. Even so, the patient may well blame the innocent prescriber.

Administration of remedies to breastfed babies

Although not a matter of routine practice, it is possible to treat a breastfed baby by administering the appropriate remedy to its mother. This effect is more likely due to the direct interaction of the general electromagnetic fields of mother and infant when in close proximity, rather than being produced via the milk (although further studies with expressed milk might confirm or refute one or other theory). It might be thought, therefore, that treating a mother who is actively breast-feeding might produce problems for her baby. This, however, is a rare consequence of the use of potentized remedies. The case with orthodox drugs and some herbal prescriptions may obviously be somewhat different.

Complex prescriptions

The purist view of prescribing suggests that only one remedy should be given at a time. Nevertheless, much good OTC prescribing is carried out with well-established mixtures, often called 'complex' or 'combination' remedies. A complex, by definition, is a mixture of remedies which have been potentized *individually*. If the various original substances were potentized together, then the Γ% values of their various molecules and ions would be somewhat different, as would, therefore, their clinical effects (see Chapter 2, *Impurities*; Chapter 3, *Remedies as fields* and *Geometric concepts*).

Most complex mixtures contain only one example of each remedy, though their selected potencies may be different, according to the intentions of the formulator (e.g. *Euphrasia* 30c, *Sabadilla* 12c, *Allium cepa* 6c). *Secretin Co.*, however (made by Ainsworths), is an unusual type of complex mixture containing a number of different potencies of one and the same remedy. On a theoretical basis, these various potencies of *Secretin* are supportable within a diluent (Lessell, 2002), but it is debatable whether the same applies *in vivo*. After administration, it would seem more likely that the various potencies are blended together to produce a single hologram of average intensity. A rather similar situation arises when two or more individual remedies in a complex contain imprints of the same ion – e.g. Na^+ in *Natrum muriaticum* and *Natrum sulphuricum* – but at different levels of potency.

Placebos

Placebos are generally unmedicated solid forms of any variety. Their main use should be in controlled clinical trials. However, some practitioners who administer only infrequent therapeutic dosages to the patient (e.g. once per month), favour them as an interim measure, if only to appease the patient's psyche. These days, except in the treatment of hypochondria or in patients who respond to suggestion alone, such a practice is to be considered as an unwarranted deception, and should be discouraged. Canny practitioners, not wishing to use the word 'placebo', often substitute the abbreviation 'Sac. lac.' – meaning 'Saccharum lactis', i.e. 'unmedicated lactose'.

Of course, there are many opponents of homeopathy who believe that our remedies merely work as placebos. Indeed, anyone who watched the BBC2 *Horizon* programme of November 2002 might have been influenced in this direction. Here we saw the positive results of both clinical trials (by Reilly of the Glasgow Homeopathic Hospital in Scotland) and *in vitro* studies (by Benveniste from France and Ennis of the University of Belfast) balanced against an apparently thorough *in vitro* trial (The Royal Society plus James Randi – 'The Great Randi') with negative results (see www.bbc.co.uk/science/horizon). How are we to understand this?

In the first place, a homeopathic remedy does not generally have the same biological properties as the drug from which it is derived. We all know that when we give *Belladonna* (according to proper indications) to a red-faced febrile patient, pallor is produced rather than plethora. So why should we expect – as the *Horizon* programme set out to test – potentized *Histamine* to act like histamine itself? The answer of course, is that we should not – except in *rare* instances (see Chapter 3, *Remedies as fields*). These relatively scarce events are certainly seen in experimental or sporadic provings (see above, *Adverse effects of potentized remedies*; also Chapter 1, *More about cause and cure*). However, they are by no means routine, and depend, in part, on the sensitivity of the subject. What Benveniste and Ennis (Ennis and Brown, 2001) appear to have demonstrated is thus an inconstant phenomenon, and one which is not readily replicated. Had it been otherwise, my faith in my own theories of homeopathy would have been shaken (rather than stirred) by the results of the BBC programme. So, congratulations *Horizon* on the – albeit unwitting – demonstration of one important homeopathic principle!

In the second place, we cannot ignore the influence of the observer in homeopathic trials. It has been said – and I was initially reluctant to accept the fact – that the more stringent the test conditions, the more likely a null result. That is to say, the more you deny observers knowledge of what is being tested, the greater the probability of a negative outcome. This observer effect is not so much (if at all) apparent in the routine pharmaceutical production of remedies, but in their action on the living organism, be it plant, animal or cell. It would seem that for a remedy to exert an effect on an organism, there must be also injected some form of subconscious or conscious thought, which we may term 'positive intention'. *This is quite independent of any psychological placebo effect.* Intention acts as a catalyst to a cascade of events triggered by a homeopathic remedy. Though the remedy is something physical, in that it is a specially contoured 'piece' of electromagnetism (see Chapter 3), its interaction with the general electromagnetic field of an organism (or group of cells *in vitro*) appears to require intervention of the human psyche. *In this respect, a potentized remedy is quite different from a material drug, which does not require such a catalyst for its action.*

From what I have said, it is not too difficult to see that there is also a thing called 'negative intention'. This may be imposed on any experimental investigation by the experimenters themselves, or by persons remote from the experiment but who know that it is taking place. Physical presence is not a prerequisite for either positive or negative influences on scientific trials. And it is the summation of all the positive and negative intentions of the persons concerned with the experiment which will partially determine the result. Intention, however, must be focused or tuned. Some are better at doing this than others. A powerful 'negative intender', such as The Great Randi, can work all sorts of mischief with the subtle process of remedial effect. Great 'positive intenders', like Reilly perhaps, can perform opposite 'miracles'. Some, like Benveniste, Ennis, or their assistants, may induce (albeit subconsciously) the electromagnetic field of cellular preparations to reverse the gestalt of the remedy, so that it produces effects similar to those of the drug of origin; and the same may happen with people directing or carrying out experimental provings of substances in potency. Many people require a more precise definition of the material to be tested before they can exert either catalysis or inhibition of biological effect, and the more stringent the trial, the less is their influence.

Of course, all this sounds quite mystical. However, it has strong support in the tenets of quantum mechanics, which hold that the outcome of a quantum experiment is partially determined by the observer. Even beyond this, the quantum idea that the structure of the universe depends on the intercommunication of every particle and object suggests that such conscious or subconscious influences of mind over matter are a stark reality – and certainly so in such subtle and delicate matters as the homeopathic effect. The basis for this most strange process is discussed in some detail in the ARH Monograph, *A New Physics of Homeopathy* (Lessell, 2002: Ch. 3).

Glossary of physicochemical terms

'Nothing in science has any value to society if it is not communicated'

Anne Roe (1953) *The Making of a Scientist*

Internal cross-references given in **bold italics**.

Agonism Effects caused by an *agonist*.
Agonist A substance which activates a *receptor*.
Allopathy Orthodox medicine.
Amino acid Any of a group of water-soluble molecules with the general formula R–CH(NH$_2$)COOH, where R may be hydrogen or an organic group.
Amino group –NH$_2$.
Angiotensins Endogenous *peptides* which raise blood pressure.
Anion A negatively charged ion.
Antagonism Effects caused by an *antagonist*.
Antagonist A substance which inactivates a *receptor*.
Arachidonic acid An *unsaturated* 20-carbon fatty acid necessary for the biosynthesis of *prostaglandins* and *leukotrienes*.
Autacoids Local *hormones*. These include: *histamine*, *serotonin*, endogenous *peptides* (e.g. *angiotensins*), *prostaglandins*, *leukotrienes* and *cytokines*.
Benzene (aromatic) ring An hexagonal ring of carbon atoms.
Binding The positional stabilization of a substance at a *receptor* site, involving *docking* and *locking*.
Biophotons *Photons* produced by living organisms.
Blocking *Antagonism*.

Glossary of physicochemical terms

Capacitance The ability to store electric charge or *energy of potentization*.
Capacitor Something possessing *capacitance*.
Carbonyl group >C=O.
Carboxyl group –COOH.
Casimir effect A very small force of attraction (sometimes repulsion) produced when two bodies are very closely approximated (i.e. a few *nanometres*), and caused by *virtual photons* of the *zero point field*.
Cation A positively charged ion.
Cellulose A *polysaccharide* consisting of a long unbranched chain of glucose molecules.
Chitin A *polysaccharide* chain composed of N-acetylglucosamine residues.
Clathrate An enclosure or cage compound, where one molecule is trapped within a lattice composed of other molecules.
Clathrate hydrate A *clathrate*, where the cage or lattice is formed by clustered water molecules held together by *hydrogen bonds*.
Coherent radiation Electromagnetic radiation in which different waves have a constant phase relationship (i.e. with peaks and troughs always similarly spaced). Because *photons* may also be regarded as waves, so we may talk of 'coherent photons'.
Colloid A solution (or suspension) in which the solute is present in the solvent in the form of charged particles 10^{-9}–10^{-6}m in length, rather than as single molecules or ions.
Covalent bond A chemical bond formed by sharing of valence (valency) electrons, rather than by transfer.
Cyclic compound One which has a ring of atoms in its molecule.
Cytokines Large heterogeneous group of *proteins* with diverse functions, including regulation of the immune system.
Desensitization, receptor A reduction of *receptor* sensitivity of rapid onset.
Digital Discontinuous representation.
Dilution The volume of solvent in which a given amount of solute is dissolved.

Dipole A pair of separated electric charges of opposite polarity.
Docking The purely geometric *binding* of a substance to a *receptor*.
Down-regulation A reduction of *receptor* response which develops more slowly than that associated with *desensitization*.
Drug Any chemical substance, synthetic or otherwise, and of known or unknown composition, which is used as a medicament to prevent or cure disease.
Electrostatic interaction The attraction of molecules by virtue of their electric charges.
Enantiomers Optical *isomers*, in which one isomer rotates the plane of plane-polarized light in one direction, whilst the other does so by the same amount in the other.
Endotoxin A *toxin* released from bacteria only when they die or disintegrate.
Energy of potentization An unknown form of energy responsible for fuelling the transfer of geometric information from solute to solvent.
Enzyme A *protein* which catalyses biochemical reactions.
Exotoxin A *toxin* secreted by bacteria into the surrounding medium.
Field A region of space (or space–time) containing specifically defined energy rather than matter (e.g. the gravitational field, magnetic field, *zero point field*).
Field, receptor A *receptor* considered for theoretical purposes as an energetic *field* rather than as a material entity.
Growth factors *Proteins* which regulate the production of blood cells.
Histamine Formed from the *amino acid* histidine, a substance released during allergic reaction.
Hologram An optical interference pattern produced by illuminating an object with *coherent radiation* in a special manner. The image of the object is projected in 3D when the hologram is subsequently illuminated with coherent radiation.
Hormone A substance which is manufactured and secreted into the bloodstream in very small quantities by an endocrine gland

or a specialized nerve cell, and which regulates the function of a specific organ or tissue.

Hydrogen bond A type of *electrostatic interaction* (*dipole*–dipole attraction) between electronegative atoms in one molecule and hydrogen atoms bound to electronegative atoms in another.

Hydrophobic interaction The clustering of *non-polar molecules* in aqueous solution, where they have been squeezed together by *polar* water *molecules*.

Hydroxyl group –OH.

Interaction Chemical bonding.

Ionic (electrovalent) bond A chemical bond formed by the transfer of electrons from one element to another.

Isomers Chemical compounds which have the same molecular formulae, but different molecular structures or different spatial arrangements of atoms.

Leukotrienes *Lipids* derived from *arachidonic acid* produced during inflammation, leading to smooth muscle contraction and swelling (important in the generation of asthma).

Ligand, pharmacological A molecule or ion, or part of a molecule or ion, which binds to a *receptor* site (see also *binding*).

Lipid Any of a large number of organic compounds occurring in living organisms which are insoluble in water but soluble in organic solvents.

Locking The chemical bonding of a substance at a *receptor* site.

Macromolecule Any large biological molecule.

Molar concentration A measure of the number of molecules or ions of solute contained in a given volume of solution, and expressed as moles/unit vol.

Molecular dipole An unbalanced distribution of electrical charge across a molecule, giving one side a more positive charge, and the other a more negative charge.

Nanometre $1 nm = 10^{-9} m$.

Neurotransmitter A substance which mediates the transmission of the nerve impulse across a synapse (e.g. adrenaline/epinephrine, noradrenaline/norepinephrine, acetylcholine).

Non-polar molecules Symmetrical molecules without *molecular dipole*.

Nucleic acid A complex compound consisting of chains of *nucleotides*. There are two types: DNA and RNA.

Nucleotide An organic compound consisting of a nitrogen-containing pyrimidine or purine base linked to a sugar – either deoxyribose or ribose – and a phosphate group.

Open chain A chain of atoms which arises when the ring of a *cyclic compound* is split.

Peptide bonds Bonds formed by the reaction between adjacent *carboxyl* and *amino groups* with the elimination of water.

Peptides Any of a group of organic compounds comprising two or more *amino acids* linked by *peptide bonds*.

Pharmaceutics The procurement, processing and chemistry of *drugs*.

Pharmacodynamics The study of the action of *drugs* on the living organism.

Pharmacokinetics The study of the action of the living organism on *drugs*.

Photons Energetic particles with zero rest mass, each consisting of a quantum of electromagnetic radiation.

Polar molecule A molecule with a *molecular dipole*.

Polypeptide A *peptide* composed of ten or more amino acids.

Polysaccharide A carbohydrate composed of a long chain of simple *sugar* (monosaccharide) molecules.

Projection The production of a 3D image from a *hologram* by its illumination with *coherent radiation*.

Prostaglandins *Regulatory* substances (*lipids*) derived from *arachidonic acid*.

Proteins Polymers of *amino acids* with important biological roles.

Receptor (chemical) A *macromolecule* which binds a *drug*, *toxin* or endogenous *ligand*, and initiates a cascade of physiological consequences (see also *binding; field, receptor*).

Regulatory Having the property of regulating normal bodily function.

Remedy The preferred name for a *drug* given homeopathically.

Saturated compound A compound having only single *covalent bonds* in its molecule.
Serotonin 5-hydroxytryptamine (5-HT). Derived from the *amino acid* tryptophan, it affects the diameter of the blood vessels and acts as a *neurotransmitter*.
Set Any collection of objects or numbers.
Shearing The forced juxtaposition of two molecular or ionic entities of the same electrical polarity, followed by their forced distraction in a direction at right angles to the line of repulsion.
Shielding A type of *blocking*.
Spagyric Alchemical.
Stereoisomerism Where *isomers* have the same formula and functional groups, but differ in the spatial arrangement of those groups.
Subset Any object or subgroup of objects contained within a *set*.
Sugars A group of water-soluble carbohydrates of relatively low molecular weight, with a sweet taste.
Sulphydryl (thiol/mercapto) group –SH.
Toxin A chemical agent which has the ability to poison a living organism.
Unsaturated compound A compound which has double or triple *covalent bonds* in its molecule.
Van der Waals' forces Weak forces generated between two molecules in close proximity. They probably result primarily from the *Casimir effect*, but are accompanied by secondary *electrostatic interactions*.
Virtual photons *Photons* which are not directly observable, but which have a presumed or theoretical existence in terms of observable effect.
Water of crystallization Water in fixed association with a molecule, and intimately involved in its ability to form specific types of crystal.
Zero point field A universal energy *field* which exists even at absolute zero, and can probed by the *Casimir effect*.

Sources of information and supply

There are numerous fine sources, but here are a few with which to begin:

Ainsworths Homoeopathic Pharmacy
36 New Cavendish Street
London W1M 7LH, England
Tel.: 020 7935 5330; Fax: 020 7486 4313
www.ainsworths.com

Helios Homoeopathic Pharmacy
97 Camden Road, Tunbridge Wells
Kent TN1 2QR, England
Tel.: 01892 536393/537254; Fax: 01892 546850

Homeopathic Educational Services
2124 Kittredge Street
Berkeley, CA 94704, USA
Tel.: (510) 649 0294/(800) 359 9051; Fax: (510) 649 1955
mail@homeopathic.com

Hahnemann Laboratories Inc.
1940 Fourth Street
San Rafael, CA 94901, USA
Tel.: 1 888 4 ARNICA/1 888 427 6422; Fax: 1 415 451 6981

Brauer Biotherapies (Pty) Ltd
Para Road
Adelaide 5000, Australia
Tel.: (0)8 8563 2932; Fax: (0)8 8563 3398

References

Anagnostatos, G.S., Pissis, P., Viras, K., Soutzidou, M. (1998) 'Theory and experiments on high dilutions', in E. Ernst and E.G. Hahn (eds) *Homoeopathy: A Critical Appraisal.* Oxford, Butterworth Heinemann: 153–66.

Benveniste, J. (1994) 'Further biological effects induced by ultra high dilutions: inhibition by a magnetic field', in P.C. Endler and J. Schulte (eds) *Ultra High Dilution.* Dordrecht, Kluwer Academic: 35.

BHP (1882) *British Homoeopathic Pharmacopoeia* (3rd edn). London, British Homoeopathic Society and E. Gould.

Boericke, W. (1927) *Pocket Manual of Homoeopathic Materia Medica.* (Reprint.) Philadelphia, Boericke & Runyon.

Ennis, M. and Brown, V. (2001) 'Flow-cytometric analysis of basophil activation: inhibition by histamine at conventional and homeopathic concentrations', *Inflammation Research*, 50: S47–48.

FHP (1982) *French Homeopathic Pharmacopoeia.* Supplement to: *Pharmacopée Francaise* (10th edn). Paris, L'Adrapharm.

GHP (1990) *German Homeopathic Pharmacopoeia (Homöopathisches Arzneibuch).* Frankfurt, Deutscher Apotheker Verlag/Govi Verlag.

Gibson Miller, R. (2002) *Relationship of Remedies.* (Reprint.) New Delhi, B. Jain.

Hahnemann, S. (1797a) 'Einige Arten anhaltender und nachlassender Fieber (Some kinds of continued and remittent fevers)', *Journal der practischen Arzneykunde und Wundarzneykunst* (Herausgeber: C.W. Hufeland), V, 1: 22–51.

Hahnemann, S. (1797b) 'Einige periodische Krankheiten und Septimanen (Some periodic and weekly diseases)', *Journal der practischen Arzneykunde und Wundarzneykunst* (Herausgeber: C.W. Hufeland), V, 1: 52–59.

Hahnemann, S. (1845) *The Chronic Diseases: Their Specific Nature and Homoeopathic Treatment.* Vol. I. (J.H. Hempel, trans.) New York, W.M. Radde.

Haisch, B., Rueda, A., Puthoff, H.E. (1997) 'Physics of the zero point field: implications for inertia, gravitation and mass', *Speculations in Science and Technology,* 20: 99–114.

Hughes, R. and Dake, J.P. (1886) *A Cyclopaedia of Drug Pathogenesy.* Vol. I. (Reprint.) New Delhi, World Homoeopathic Links.

Hughes, R. and Dake, J.P. (1888) *A Cyclopaedia of Drug Pathogenesy.* Vol. II. (Reprint.) New Delhi, World Homoeopathic Links.

Katzung, B.G. (2001) *Basic and Clinical Pharmacology.* (International edition.) New York, Lange.

Kayne, S.B. (1997) *Homoeopathic Pharmacy: An Introduction and Handbook.* London, Churchill Livingstone.

Lessell, C.B. (1994). *The Infinitesimal Dose.* Saffron Walden, C.W. Daniel.

Lessell, C.B. (2001) *The Complementary Formulary: A Guide for Prescribers.* Oxford, Butterworth Heinemann.

Lessell, C.B. (2002) *A New Physics of Homeopathy.* Leigh-on-Sea, Alliance of Registered Homeopaths (www.a-r-h.org).

McTaggart, L. (2001) *The Field: The Quest for the Secret Force of the Universe.* London, Harper Collins.

Mohideen, U. and Roy, A. (1998) 'Precision measurement of the Casimir force from 0.1 to 0.9 μm', *Physics Review Letters,* 81: 4549–52.

Murphy, R. (1993) *Homeopathic Medical Repertory.* Pagosa Springs, Hahnemann Academy of North America.

Nash, E.B. (2002) *Leaders in Homoeopathic Therapeutics.* (Reprint.) New Delhi, B. Jain.

Puthoff, H.E. (1990) 'Everything for nothing', *New Scientist,* 127: 52–55.

Samal, S. and Geckeler, K.E. (2001) 'Unexpected solute aggregation in water on dilution', *Chemical Communications,* 21: 2224–25.

Speight, P. (1991) *A Study Course in Homeopathy.* Saffron Walden, C.W. Daniel.

Index

acute disease 95, 112, 113
administration
   dosage 106, 107, 109–11
   of LM potencies 111
   for sensitive individuals 109, 116
aggravation 21, 96–8, 99
agonism 78–80, 81, 82, 87, 92
   and dosage 88–9
   partial 79
agonist 78, 85, 91, 92
alcohol 33–4, 73, 107, 111
   and drop size 31
   in liquid phase potentization 51
   and mother tinctures 35, 36
   and viscosity 50–1
   see also ethanol
allergens 87
allopathy 2, 25, 74, 88, 104
amino acids 91
amplification sites 109, 115
anaesthesia 87–8, 115
angiotensins 77
anions 100
   see also ions
antagonism 78–80, 81, 82, 92
   functional 80
antagonist 78
anthroposophical procedure 50, 51
apparatus
   cleansing of 62
   preparatory vessels 70–1
   see also vials
Arnica 11, 18, 87–8, 90–1
aromatic substances 114–15

Arsenicum 92–3
autacoid 77, 88, 90, 94

Bach Flower Remedies 66, 69, 111
Bacillinum 19
Belladonna 2, 16, 118
benzene (aromatic) ring 40
binding 77–8
Biochemic Tissue Salts 111
biophotons 73
blocking 85–6, 87–8, 90, 91
bodies, foreign 115
Boericke, W 15
boiling 69
breast-feeding 116
bruising 90
bubbling 63–5

Calcarea fluorica 93
capacitance 49, 66
capacitor 48–9
capillary tube 32
carbonyl groups 40, 41
Casimir effect 80–2, 83, 85, 101–2
   and mercury 92
cations 93–4, 99
   see also ions
cellulose 42, 53
centesimal dilution 29, 30, 44
Chamomilla 6
chirality 82, 101
chitin 40
chronic disease 11, 12, 95, 98, 112, 113
chronic miasm 19–20

classical energization 46–62
clinical proving 3
coffee 115
colloid 39, 43, 53
'competitive agonism' 88–9
complex prescriptions 98, 116–17
conjunctivitis 91
constitution of patient 10, 22
cork 31, 42
correspondence of remedies 100
covalent bond 78, 92, 93
cramps 94, 99
critical capacitance 49, 66
Cuprum aceticum 58
Cuprum metallicum 57, 58
Cuprum sulphuricum 30–1
cyclic compounds 40, 41

decimal dilution 29, 30, 44
depotentization 69–70
desensitization 88–9, 90
detoxification 88
digital information transfer 73
diluents 39–42
   exclusion 40–2
   suitable 42
dilution 28–33, 44, 49, 52
   see also serial dilution
disease
   aggravation 96–8
   chronic 11, 12, 98
   incurable 12
   patterns 86
   response 86
distillation plants 52
docking 77–8, 83, 89
dose and dosage 88–9, 103–20
   considerations 104–6
   repetition 112–13
   size of 25–6

down-regulation 89, 90
'drainage' remedies 88
drops
   characteristics of 31–2
   standard 32
drug-receptor geometric complex 82
   viewed as fields 82–3
   viewed as sets 82, 95–6
drugs 77–101
   see also remedies
dynamization 26–8, 31, 51, 73

electromagnetic energization 66–8, 83–4
   remedies 30, 101
   and sunlight 66
   via magnetic fields 68
electromagnetic field 81, 82–3
   of body 89, 94, 95–8, 115
   mother-infant interaction 116
   and positive interaction 119
electromagnetic potentization *see* electromagnetic energization
electrostatic interaction 80
enantiomers 82, 101
endotoxin 77
energization 46–63, 73
   boiling 69
   bubbling 63–5
   classical 46–62
   electromagnetic 30, 66–8, 101
   fluxion 62–3
   methods summarized 47
   prepotentization 63–5
   succussion 46–51
   trituration 52–62

energy
  fields 82–5
  and information transfer 48–9
  loss from molecular memory 107, 114
  and mode of delivery 50
  of potentization 26–8, 51, 73
enzymes 91
epilepsy 18
ethanol 39
  see also alcohol
Euphrasia officinalis 91
'exclusion' 40
exotoxin 77
experimental proving 3
externalization 21

fields 82–5
  remedies as 83–5
  see also electromagnetic field, magnetic field
fifty millesimal (LM) dilution 29, 44
  see also LM potencies
Fincke, Bernard 63
Flower Remedies 66, 69, 111
fluid levels 94
fluxion 62–3, 65
fructose 40–1
functional therapeutic potency 112

garlic 115
gases 63–5
generals 16
genus epidemicus 22
'geometric polarity reversal' 97
geometrical conformation 78–82
  as mathematical sets 82, 95–6

geometry 73, 77, 79, 99
  and complex configuration 98
  and disease patterns 86, 95–8
  of multiple sets 98
  and physiological effects 98–9
glass 70–1, 106, 107, 114
glucose 40–1
growth factor 77

haemorrhage 90, 91
Hahnemann, Samuel 28, 30, 75, 76
  and dosage 88
  and mother tinctures 32, 33, 38, 39
  seminal works 4–5, 25, 27
  and trituration 52, 53–6, 59–62
Hepar sulph. 18
Hering's Law 20–1
histamine 77, 118
Histamine 118
hologram 73, 74, 84
homeopathic trials 118–19
hormones 77, 85
hydrogen bonding 78, 81
hydroxyl group 40

imagery and images 73–4
imprinting 26
  and atmospheric gases 62–3
  and concentration 43
  and electromagnetic phenomena 66–8
  erasure of 69–70
  and information transfer 114
  and ionization 40
  as 'mural phenomenon' 42
  and photons 68
  and serial dilution 65
  solid and liquid compared 63
  see also molecular memory

impurities 42–6
  lack of influence 44
  in trituration 59
inert materials 26, 28
information loss 107
information transfer 48–9, 58
  geometrical 73
  intermittent 84
  and laws of probability 84–5
  see also imprinting, molecular memory
insoluble materials 52–3
intensification 26
interactions 115
intolerances 2, 111
iodine 36
ionic (electrovalent) bond 40, 45–6, 78, 93–4
ions 40, 45–6, 93–4, 99, 100, 117
isomerisation 41
isomers 41
isopathy 87

Kali phosphoricum 93
keynotes 16–18
Korsakov's method 31, 62

lactose 52, 73, 111
  insolubility 53, 56
  as standard diluent 39
  and trituration 33, 40, 41
Latin 2
Law of Similars 2, 25, 26, 74–6, 102
leading symptoms 16–18
ligand, pharmacological 77–8, 79
liquid potencies 106–7

LM potencies 33–5
  administered 'wet' 111
  preparation of 33–5, 44
locking 78, 89

maceration 35, 36
macromolecule 77, 92
Magnesia phosphorica 93, 94
magnetic field 68, 69, 70, 82–3
  disturbed in living body 95–8
  potency or strength 100
  see also electromagnetic field, electromagnetic energization
magnetic pattern, viewed in terms of set geometry 95–6
Magnetis polus australis 101
materia medica 3, 15–16, 18, 19
Medorrhinum 19
memory *see* molecular memory
mentals 16
Mercurius 91–2, 93
Mercurius solubilis 6, 13, 16
miasm 19–20
microscopy 57, 58
minor ingredients 44–5
mismatch 22
modalities 7
molecular memory 26–8, 40, 73
  and atmospheric gases 62–3
  loss of energy 107, 114
  and water ionization 42
  see also imprinting
mortars 71
mother tinctures 35–9
  administration of 106, 107
  and alcohol concentration 36
  preparation of 35–6
  sell-by date 70

strength of 45
symbols for 38–9
variation in 36
multiple subsets 98
Murphy, R *Homeopathic Medical Repertory* 13

Nash, E B 18
Natrum 99
Natrum muriaticum 10, 45–6, 58, 93, 94, 117
Natrum sulphuricum 18, 46, 117
negative intention 119
neurotransmitter 77
nomenclature and labelling 2
nosodes 2, 19, 87, 113
nucleic acids 77

observer 118–19
onions 115
open chain 41
opponents of homeopathy 118–20

particulars 16
pathogenesis 3
pathological action 6
pathological simillimum *see* simillimum
patient 7–10, 113
peppermint 115
peptides 91
percolation 35, 37
pharmaceutics 73
pharmacodynamics 73
pharmacokinetics 73
Phosphorus 36, 98–9
photons 68, 73, 74, 82
   photonic energy 80, 81
   virtual 68, 80, 82

Pinkus Potentizer 62
placebos 117–18
plant material 35–9
   alcohol used 36
   converted to mother tinctures 35–6
   lack of uniformity 36
   and liquid phase potentization 39
   press 38
'plussing' 106
polar molecule 48, 78, 97
polarity reversal 97
polychrests 3, 98–9
polypeptides 77, 91
polysaccharides 40
positive intention 119
potency 2, 21–2, 101
   and dilution 33
   and dosage 104, 112
   high 85, 115–16
   of magnetic field 100
   and therapeutic response 112, 113
potentization 26–8, 31, 51, 73
   machines 62, 67, 68
pregnancy 21
preparatory vessels 70–1
prepotentization 63–5, 66
prescribing
   by causation 18
   complex 22–3, 116–17
   constitutional 7–10, 12
   pathological 7–10, 11–12
   suitable basis for 15
   and symptoms 6–7
   and thermal sensitivity 13–15
prescriptions, complex 22–3, 98, 116–17
projection 73–4, 84

prostaglandin 77
proteins 77, 91
proving 21, 22
   clinical or sporadic 3, 116
   experimental 3
psora 20

Q *see* LM potencies
quantum mechanics 119–20

rash 21
receptor-mediated action 77–93
receptors 77–93
   agonism and antagonism 78–80
   and allergens 87
   blocking 85–6, 87–8, 90–1
   and Casimir effect 80–2
   docking and locking 77–8, 89
   effect of remedies 85
   as energy fields 82–5
   and geometric conformation 82
   and laws of probability 84–5
   as mathematical sets 82
   occupancy 90
   selective nature 78
   shielding 85–6, 87, 90–1
   site pharmacology 101–2
   and toxic effect 92
   and van der Waals' forces 80–2
   and viral remedies 87
remedies
   action of 72–102
   adverse effects of 109, 115–16
   biological properties 118
   direct and indirect action 94–5
   and dose repetition 113
   duration of action 88–9
   as fields 83–5, 95
   interactions 115
   and ionic charges 74
   and multiple subsets 98
   non-receptor-mediated 93–101
   and patient constitution 7–10
   precautions when taking 114–15
   production/manufacture of 24–71
      and mode of delivery 50
   quantities 89
   receptor-mediated 77–93
   repetition 85
   selection of 1–23
      and constitutional prescribing 111–12
      and modalities 7
      provings 3
      and simillimum 3–6, 10–11
      and symptoms 6–7
      see also prescribing
repertorization 13–15
repertory 11, 12–13
   and symptoms 12
   use of 18, 19
repetition of dose 21–2
response 112, 113
rubrics 12–13

Saccharum lactis 117
scarlet fever 2
Schüssler, Wilhelm 111
Secretin Co. 117
sedimentation 106
sensitivity of patient 113
serial dilution 49, 52
   and fluxion 62
   and imprinting 65
   scales of 28–33, 73
      centesimal 29, 30, 44, 73
      decimal 29, 30, 44, 73

defined 28–9
and energy 50
fifty millesimal (LM or Q) 29, 44, 73
and trituration 56
sets and set geometry 82, 85, 95, 96
shearing 48, 50
shielding 85–6, 87–8, 90, 91
Silicea 100, 115
Similia Principle 2, 25, 26, 74–6, 102
similior 22–3
simillimum 22, 101
and constitutional prescribing 11
and pathological action 3–6, 10–11
skin rash 21
Skinner, Thomas 63, 64
sodium 45–6, 93, 99, 100, 117
sodium chloride 45–6
Sol 101
solid forms 71, 107, 108
converted to liquid 59–62
spagyric sigil 38
sporadic proving 3
steel containers 107
Steiner, Rudolf 50
stereoisomerism 82, 101
storage 106, 107
subjects, sensitive 85, 109, 116
subset 83, 85, 95, 96, 98, 99
succussion 30, 42–3, 46–51, 106
and impurities 42
machines 48, 49
numbers per dilution 50
procedures 47
sugars 41
sulphur 91
Sulphur 20, 98–9

sulphydryl (thiol/mercapto) group 91–3
sunlight 66, 68
susceptible typology 10
sycosis 20
symptomatology 6, 94
symptoms
aggravation 90, 98, 99, 115–16
concomitant 7
order of clearing 20–1
in prescribing 6–7, 22
syphilis 20

tap water 45
therapeutic index 6
use of 18, 19, 22
thermal sensitivity 13–15
toxicity reduction 26–8
toxins 77, 78–80, 86, 88, 94
transfer of information *see* information transfer
trituration 43–6, 52–62
dilutions 53–8
and insoluble materials 52–3
machines 53, 54–5, 56
microscopy 57, 58
procedure detailed 59–62
and remedy administration 111
tuberculosis 19
Type I action 77–93, 101, 102
Type II action 93–101

ultraviolet light 66, 69–70
unsaturated compound 40

Vacuum Device 65
van der Waals' forces 78, 79, 80–2
VDU 68, 101

vials 48–9, 70–1, 106, 107, 114
   and impurities 30, 42
   see also apparatus
viral remedies (viral nosodes) 87
virtual photons 68, 80, 82

water 39, 42

x-rays 68, 69, 70

zero point field 80, 81